With the compliments of
Tony Williams. May 23RD. 1991.

MEDICAL AUDIT
AND GENERAL PRACTICE

MEDICAL AUDIT
AND GENERAL PRACTICE

Edited by

MARSHALL MARINKER, FRCGP

Director, The MSD Foundation, London

Published for The MSD Foundation
by the British Medical Journal
Tavistock Square, London WC1H 9JR

First published 1990
Reprinted 1991

British Library Cataloguing in Publication Data

Medical audit and general practice.
1. Patients. Care. Planning
I. Marinker, Marshall
362.172

ISBN 0–7279–0295–4

Typeset and printed in Great Britain
by Latimer Trend & Company Ltd, Plymouth

Contents

Preface

Medical audit is a promising means to an essential end—improving the quality of medical care that the patient receives. A commitment to medical audit has now been expressed by the major professional bodies concerned with clinical medicine in the National Health Service. None the less, anxieties remain. Will medical audit be simply a device for controlling the contract between the doctor and the state? What will be audited? Who will determine this? Who will write the standards? To whom are the auditors accountable? What will be the consequences for the professionalism of doctors, for the independence of the practice, for the standards of care that the patient will receive?

This book is designed for general practitioners who wish to embark on medical audit. It is concerned not only with the mechanisms of audit in general practice but also with its philosophy and intentions. Most of the authors are principals in general practice. They have described an approach to medical audit that is rooted in the experience of general practice. However stringently the present or future contracts of general practitioners are monitored by the health care authorities appropriate standards of care must be identified, composed, and monitored effectively by those with direct responsibility for the care of patients.

Rudolph Klein,[1] commenting on the larger transformations of British society, wrote that in the 1980s the relationship between the professions and the public shifted from one based on status and trust to one based on contract. Nevertheless, in the past the achievements and success of British general practice have resulted not from the wording of contracts or the imposition of control but from the free exercise of professional good conscience. This book seeks to build on this professional good conscience by explaining the role of medical audit in the future development of each practice and of general practice as a professional discipline.

The intention has been to provide practical guidelines without

ix

being prescriptive: to leave room for the diversity, creativity, and energy which have ensured the best of practice and which, with the help of medical audit, can achieve so much more.

MARSHALL MARINKER
July 1990

1 Klein R. From status to contract: the transformation of the British medical profession. In: *Proceedings of Anglo-American Symposium on health care provision under financial constraint: a decade of change.* (University of North Carolina, 1990). In press.

Acknowledgments

It is a pleasure to express my thanks to so many friends and collaborators who have made this book possible. Foremost, I want to thank William Anderson, who acted as managing editor. Coming from a distinguished background in science education and the arts, he approached this fresh territory of medical audit with a proper academic mix of enthusiasm and scepticism. All the authors have benefited from his gentle questioning of their intentions, and the firm editing that followed.

Ian Bogle, Sir Michael Drury, and Bill Styles joined me on the editorial advisory team. They gave unstinting support to what became a fruitful and enjoyable collaboration. They would wish to join me in stating that the support from authors has been exemplary: copy was produced before deadlines expired and the pain of redrafting, and sometimes redrafting again, endured with forbearance and good humour.

The Department of Health was generous in making a financial grant towards the production of the book and true to its word in giving the editors free rein. Neil Poppmacher and Dorothy Sharp of the *British Medical Journal* have given great help and sound advice.

Finally, I wish to record my sincerest thanks to the staff of The MSD Foundation: Graham Ball, who co-ordinated the administration, and Sarah Poyner, who so patiently and accurately produced the typescript.

MARSHALL MARINKER

Principles

MARSHALL MARINKER

Creativity and error

Medical science, in common with all other sciences, depends on a balance, a congruity, and a collaboration between creativity and critique. If clinical medicine is to be scientific in its orientation and honesty the general practitioner must be creative in his search for good standards of practice and his own sternest critic in searching for error.

The habit of truth is central to scientific endeavour. Perhaps the most powerful tool of modern science has been the pursuit of the null hypothesis. Here the task of the scientist is to submit what he believes to be the truth to the most searching attack that evidence and logic can mount. He attempts to prove that what he has found is simply a chance event or random relationship, which has no general relevance or validity. The search for error is the crucial expression of the habit of truth. Yet much in medical education and medical practice teaches us to associate error with blame, and blame with shame and punishment. No wonder that we have little appetite to search for error.

It is possible to be active or passive in our efforts to suppress the truth or to fail to recognise it. I can hide the fact that I have prescribed a harmful medication, or failed to understand or act appropriately on the evidence to hand. That is active deceit. Of course my professional conscience will prick me. I may also fear the shame of discovery more than I fear the pain of confessing my fault. But at least my deceit is conscious and amenable to challenge.

But I can also fail to recognise error simply by refusing to search for it, by being over zealous in my compliance with current belief. Much of my own education at medical school encouraged this professional good conduct. This is passive deceit, and it is much more dangerous than active deceit. It stunts the growth of

1

knowledge; it strengthens authority and it paralyses creativity. And it does all this silently, because the professional conscience is anaesthetised by habit and conformity.

McKintyre and Popper[1] called for a new ethics of medical practice in which error would be valued, cherished even, as a major source of learning. They write:

In monitoring medical care tolerance is essential and in the search for mistakes there should be no denigration of others nor any condemnation associated with the process of peer review. It would be morally wrong and would deter doctors from taking part. The goal must be educational and practical: it must be linked to the improvement of all doctors and not to the punishment of those who err. Only with such an ethos can we establish a new type of confidence: that mutual criticism is not personal and pejorative but that it springs from a mutual respect and a desire to improve the lot of patients.

As therapies become more powerful the public protects itself with more ambitious and punishing litigation. Those who hold the budgets for medical care (whether a government department or a private insurance company) demand tighter and tighter contractual controls over the performance of doctors. In this sense "error" and "deviations from contractual norms" may be dangerously confused. Medical audit is a means of searching for error. If it becomes only a tool for monitoring deviations from contractual norms it will have little to do with science and quality. McKintyre and Popper look forward to a robust independent profession so open to self critical analysis that the public will have little need for litigation, and the government will have less cause to impose tight contracts.

The search for error is part of the search for continuous improvement in health care. Berwick[2] examines the theory of quality improvement in industry and applies this to the practice of medicine. He writes:

... a test result lost, a specialist who cannot be reached, a missing requisition, a misinterpreted order, duplicate paperwork, a vanished record, a long wait for the CT scan, an unreliable on-call system—these are all-too-familiar examples of waste, rework, complexity, and error in the doctor's daily life. ... For the average doctor, quality fails when systems fail.

Berwick contrasts two approaches to the search for error. He calls the first the "theory of bad apples": here the approach is punitive, and there are overtones of "recertification" or "deterrents" or "litigation." Of this approach he writes: "In fact, practically no system of measurement—at least none that measures people's performance—is robust enough to survive the fear of those who are measured."

The second approach that he describes is widely used in Japanese industry. It is called *kaizen*. In medical care *kaizen* would mean that every health care worker involved in a particular system would be encouraged and educated to improve performance. In place of punishment there would be a sense of discovery, pride, and achievement brought about by creative leadership. That is what we see in the best of British general practice today, and this book is written in the hope and expectation of encouraging just such an approach.

Coming to terms

In the literature of medical audit each author creates his own definition of the term, and each definition varies subtly from all those which went before. Let me then propose my own. *Medical audit is the attempt to improve the quality of medical care by measuring the performance of those providing that care, by considering the performance in relation to desired standards, and by improving on this performance.* The reader will be immediately aware that every term used in my definition gives rise to further questions, rather than explanations. The opening two chapters of this book are concerned with the exploration of some of the questions raised and with a search for some further explanations.

The term medical audit has been with us for two decades. During that time it has given rise to a burgeoning literature. A search through this literature reveals a number of other terms, used either as synonyms or to identify closely allied concepts. Terms such as "standard setting," "performance review," "peer review," and "quality assurance" have been coined to explain medical audit, to soften or sharpen the image, or to apologise for it.

An exponential growth of papers and books on any subject is more often a sign of hope, enthusiasm, and uncertainty than of success, benefit, and proof. Further, the enthusiasm for medical audit shown not only by clinicians and medical academics but also by politicians and Treasury civil servants may suggest that, while all the proponents may know what they are talking about, they are not necessarily talking about the same thing. Indeed, as this book will reveal, the implementation of medical audit embraces philosophical speculation and examination of moral values, a reinterpretation both of clinical teaching and of the logic of clinical problem solving, the numerical skills of epidemiology, the narrative skills of case discussion, and the political skills of negotiating change. All of these, at one time or another, must be employed in the course of medical audit.

Since there are no universally accepted crisp and clear definitions of the terms used, no single purpose for the use of audit, no copper bottomed guarantees (backed by hard evidence) that the game is worth the candle, what then is the rationale for this book? Clearly the authors believe strongly in the value of medical audit. This belief alone, however, would scarcely constitute a defence for writing the book. That defence must rest on other supports—from logic, from experience, and from the results of research. Medical audit should be characterised by the discipline which it serves, by medicine itself. Medicine is more than a biotechnology. It is both art and science, both philosophy and politics. The American sociologist Ashley Montague[3] wrote that medicine was neither an art nor a science in itself but rather a special sort of relationship between two people: the doctor and his patient. Unless medical audit impinges materially and beneficially on the clinical and social purpose of this relationship there will be little motivation to learn about it, to develop it, and to practise it.

Medical audit is not an end in itself. It is a tool to achieve a desired end. In fact medical audit refers to a number of tools, fashioned to achieve a number of different ends. These ends may be described as contractual, managerial, or educational. Inevitably there is an overlap between all three. Compliance with a contract is in fact a managerial imperative. All medical audit, no matter what its intentions, reveals something new to the auditor and so has educational value. None the less, it may be useful to consider the differences between the contractual intentions of medical audit and the more imaginative use of audit as a guide to better clinical practice and practice management.

Contractual intentions

Audit for the purposes of contract is centrally concerned with compliance and control. The family health service authority* (in Scotland, health board) may seek to monitor a contract that specifies a range of performances and levels of performance. Here medical audit may be used simply to provide evidence that the contract has been fulfilled, that the range and levels of performance have been attained, and therefore that appropriate payment can be made. In this form of audit no questions are raised about appropriateness, about the benefit or cost of the audit, or about the impact on the health of patients. The problems of medical audit for the purposes of contract might therefore appear to be simply mechanical. This appearance is misleading because in fact there are moral as well as technical problems to be tackled.

One important example, from the new National Health Service contract for general practitioners, will suffice. Cervical cytology is an invasive procedure. In the course of clinical problem solving there is an evident ethical duty on the part of the doctor to negotiate such invasive procedures. When such an invasive procedure is carried out not on a patient with a relevant medical problem but on a well person in the search for hidden disease this duty is made sharper and more urgent. Such negotiation would be difficult enough, even if the benefits from such screening could be securely demonstrated from scientific research. In fact, there is room for discussion and doubt.[4] The clinical significance of abnormal histology, apart from the finding of actual malignant change, remains uncertain. These so called abnormal findings may occur in up to 30% of specimens examined. There is no consensus about how to interpret them, or about what action should follow. There remain questions about cost/benefit—cost expressed not only in financial terms but in terms of the patient's anxiety and distress. To complete the list of dilemmas, the new contract rewards the general practitioner financially for obtaining high levels of compliance with the procedure, in a population of otherwise well persons.

The major difference between carrying out medical audit for the purposes of contract and carrying out audit to improve clinical care and practice management may be psychological. Contractual audit

* This is the term introduced from September 1990 to replace family practitioner committee, the term used elsewhere in the book.

may appear to be regulatory and punitive rather than developmental. None the less, it may serve as an introduction to "the real thing." Because the mechanics of selecting, handling, and interpreting the data are similar, no matter what the purposes of the auditor, these contractual audits may be regarded as simple five finger exercises: a necessary rehearsal. There is a further benefit to be gained from success in carrying out such contractual audits. Practice income can thus be maximised. Maximising practice income creates greater freedom and funds to improve the service to patients.

Audit for clinical and practice management

Medical audit is concerned with much more than fulfilling the terms of any current contract. It is concerned with questions about the range of services offered to patients; how and why these may change over time; what choices should be made about the use of limited resources; what standards of care should be aimed for and on what basis these standards will be created, judged, and revised. The role of control and compliance, so important in contractual audit, is secondary and subservient to these much more important priorities. The following tasks are required in an overall management audit strategy.

- Determining which aspects of current work are to be considered
- Describing and measuring present performance and trends
- Developing explicit standards
- Deciding what needs to be changed
- Negotiating change
- Mobilising resources for change
- Reviewing and renewing the process.

It will be clear that these seven tasks require an imaginative and creative approach to what it is that the practice is there to do. The development of general practice now demands, as never before, that partners and other members of the practice are given an opportunity to explore their ideas for the future, and to discover a strong sense of ownership of these ideas and enterprises. All the partners in a practice, and all the colleagues who work with them in the primary health care team, will be involved in one aspect or another of medical audit. All these tasks require sensitive and rigorous group work, and this is discussed further on pages 185–95.

The practice of medical audit, like the practice of clinical science, demands a mixture of creativity and critical analysis. The auditors must therefore consider, in relation to anything that they are planning to do, what resources are needed. What *information* will be necessary to monitor events? A sound principle in determining what data are required is the principle of economy of effort. All too often enthusiastic auditors set about collecting and collating almost all the data available on their chosen topic. Later there is a discussion (pages 168–84) on the sampling of data and other ways of reducing the number of facts that must be looked for and processed. Consideration of the information required leads to choice of the *necessary technology*. Increasingly, the microcomputer is becoming an indispensable tool of practice management and medical audit. Consideration must then be given to *personnel*: the various tasks of medical audit must be distributed among members of the practice in accordance with their aptitudes, their interests, and their commitment. Clear definition of tasks and responsibilities is essential, although these cannot be ascribed by dictate but must be negotiated. *Time* may be perceived by members of the practice as the most scarce resource. A realistic estimate of the time involved in medical audit is essential. Much has been written about the management of time, but time has to be "created" rather than "found." Creating time for medical audit involves a reallocation of some tasks, and perhaps the abandoning of others that have been kept going, not because they are particularly beneficial but because they are part of the practice's traditional way of working. Finally *space* must be found and allocated, and those responsible for the practice's budget must take account of the *financial cost*.

What can be measured or described?

Avedis Donabedian,[5] perhaps the most influential theorist in the field of quality assurance in health care, differentiates between three aspects of a health service: structure, process, and outcome.

Structure refers to the physical and personnel resources of an organisation. Examples would include the building, the number of rooms and their size and use; the equipment that the practice employs; the number of patients and ratio of patients to doctors; the number and categories of other staff. Structure is perhaps the easiest to measure of the three components of health care. One of the first formal approaches to medical audit in general practice, that initiated by the Joint Committee on Postgraduate Medical Training,[6] relied heavily on such measurements. The relative ease with which structure can be measured is balanced by the relative difficulty—I would rather say near impossibility—of making other than value judgments about them. These value judgments, however, are both inescapable and appropriate.

Process refers to the actions taken by all those involved in the aspect of care that is being audited. Processes would include measurements of consultation rates, the items recorded in the records, the frequency of use of particular instruments, investigations carried out or referral to other health care personnel, the number and type of drugs prescribed, and the frequency and scale of the use of all other health care resources. It will be clear that the number of processes that can be measured in relation to any particular aspect of medical care is considerable, and choices must be limited by the resources available for measurement and interpretation. The measurement of process is the most common activity in medical audit. Medical audit as defined in the general practitioners' new contract is almost exclusively concerned with the measurement of process. Most of the audits described in this book rest largely on the measurement and interpretation of items of process.

Outcome refers to the results of health care, and health care may be described as the product of the structures (the resources that are available) plus the processes (the activities of the health care workers concerned). These outcomes are expressed in terms of the patient's health status or physical or social function. Suicide and parasuicide rates might be used as an outcome measure of the success or failure of diagnosing and treating depression. School absence might be a useful outcome measure in assessing the diagnosis and management of childhood asthma.

Making judgments

Purists have argued that only an audit of outcome is worth while, that measures of structure and process are of value only if they can be shown to have a direct link with the outcome. Without the evidence of such a direct link, it is argued, it is impossible to know how either structures or processes should be changed. This purist view is certainly not supported by Donabedian, nor, I think, is it supported by logical analysis of the purposes and possibilities of medical audit.

As far as measurements of structure are concerned, value judgments may be made without too much embarrassment. Is it really necessary to demonstrate that a cold and cramped consulting room with poor sound insulation results in failures of diagnosis or deteriorations in health? The absence of an effective steriliser, a paucity of support staff, the lack of reference books in the consulting room, or of a practice library, may all be safely judged as having a negative influence on the quality of care.

Value judgments about process data rely in part on logic and common sense and in part on the results of previous good research. Both these reference points (common sense and research) although indispensable must be treated with some reserve. The common sense of one decade may appear nothing more than a passing fashion in the next. Most good research provides not only answers to clinical problems but fresh questions, a stimulus to new research, and the possibility that the previous answers will be found inadequate.

The judgments that flow from research can sometimes appear less securely anchored in hard evidence than judgments based on common sense and professional values. Fifteen years ago research suggested that in children under the age of 3 years *H influenzae* was a common cause of otitis media and therefore that penicillin V would be ineffective and a broader spectrum antibiotic should be employed. Since then much research has suggested that the use of antibiotics has little effect on the natural history of otitis media in children. A recent review article[7] suggests that perhaps after all there is a place for antibiotic therapy in the management of this condition.

Items of process like the recording of risk factors—for example, drug idiosyncracies—in the patient's notes must self evidently appear to be a good thing. Their general absence from the practice's record system may be regarded with justified anxiety. In a recent paper Howie[8] chose to regard the prescribing of an antibiotic for children with upper respiratory tract infections as an indicator of poor care. His judgment was based on the results of a great deal of research, including his own, that suggests that such antibiotic treatment is relatively ineffective. In his paper Howie makes it clear that he is making a value judgment based in part on findings from research and in part on logic and extrapolation. This honesty allows others to come to a decision about how much credence they can give to his conclusions.

Another example of the use of process measures as an indicator of the quality of care concerns the routine monitoring of blood pressure measurement in the audit population, in the search for moderate to severe hypertension, long advocated[9] as one of the benchmarks of good preventive medicine in modern general practice. This judgment is based on much research that correlated hypertension with the incidence of stroke and established the benefits of controlling this hypertension.

The rub is that while measures of outcome are intellectually satisfying they are also quite rare. There are a number of reasons for this. So many factors affect the natural history of most medical conditions that it can be difficult to say that the outcomes observed were actually brought about, or materially affected, by the structures and processes desired. Despite massive research into the surgery, radiotherapy, and chemotherapy of breast cancer, we still remain uncertain about the treatment of choice. To take another example, our knowledge of the causes, course, and management of lower back pain is so insubstantial that few would be prepared to make a firm link between the choice of therapy and the ensuing duration and severity of the symptoms.

Where good research has been able to establish firm links between process and outcome measures of process can be accepted with some confidence as indicators of quality. An example would be evidence from glycosylated haemoglobin measurements that blood sugar is being well controlled in diabetics. We know from research that end organ damage is reduced when blood sugar is well controlled by diet and medication. Glycosylated haemoglobin measurements correlate strongly with levels of blood glucose control over long periods of time.

Populations and samples

For the most part medical audit refers to the monitoring of populations. It is a golden rule of medical audit, as of all empirical research, that the greatest benefit, in terms of what is to be learnt, should be purchased for the smallest cost, in terms of the number of resources used and data collected. There may therefore be situations in which it would be both economical and morally acceptable to create a small representative sample from the total number; for example, the practice might wish to check that the records of addresses and telephone numbers of its elderly patients are valid. Here sampling may be sufficient to provide evidence of overall practice performance in this area of documentation. The relationship between the size of the sample and the confidence we can have in the results of our findings, and the ways in which valid samples may be chosen, are considered by Ian and Daphne Russell (see pages 168–84).

When medical audit is used to improve the care of certain categories of patients the sample should contain all those patients known to be suffering from the same condition. The reasons for this are self evident. Since we know from previous large population studies something about the prevalence of each condition in relation to the age/sex distribution of the practice population the finding of a lower proportion of hypertensives or diabetics or asthmatics than might have been expected would provoke the questions: "How can we improve our early diagnosis of this condition? How can we improve the efficiency of our disease register?" In this kind of audit it is important to include in the population being studied all those patients who have the condition that is being audited. The reason is a practical one: if error is detected this can be rectified for the individual patient, whose care is thus improved.

Sometimes the population being considered—whether a whole population or a sampled one—is referred to as the *denominator*. Not all denominators need to be based on the practice population, nor on a subset of the practice population characterised by the presence of a particular disease or other characteristic. It can sometimes be useful to make measurements based on a series of consultations; for example, in attempting an audit of the care of children with cough, or of adults with back pain, the practice may monitor a sequence of consultations. Here it is important to include all the events in the series. Much can be learnt from, say, 50 consecutive consultations for a particular condition or complaint. By insisting that the denominator is made up of *consecutive* events, the practice may be able to generalise from the findings. If the auditor departs from this discipline—for example, by excluding the patients seen on Wednesdays or Fridays because the practice is particularly busy or understaffed on those days—the denominator can no longer be relied upon as being unbiased, and therefore the "findings" can have little relevance.

The individual case

A quite different approach to audit is based not on the measurement of populations or of series of events but on the evaluation of *individual significant events*. Examples from clinical medicine would include an audit of sudden or unexpected deaths, emergency admissions to hospital, suicide attempts, episodes of coronary thrombosis or stroke, newly registered blindness, episodes of iatrogenic illness and mishaps. Examples from the organisation of the practice would include such matters as the failure to visit the patient at home after a request for a visit had been accepted; a failure to despatch letters or to file them, or to take action on them; failure to deliver urgent messages; breakdown of relationships between the members of the practice team; breaches of confidentiality; and so on.

The study of individual cases in an attempt to learn from mistakes and to experiment with new methods gave rise to what we now call the clinicopathological conference. This form of medical audit, with its basis in the postmortem room, has transformed the quality of clinical care in the hospital setting. A variety of clinicians, medical scientists, and others involved in the care of the patient critically examine their own performance and seek to learn from their own mistakes.

General practice has, in fact, developed a different but very strong tradition of case discussion, based on small groups. This teaching method has a central place in contemporary vocational training. Balint[10] seminars were perhaps the first and in many ways are still the most rigorous example of this method. Although the Balint approach is primarily concerned with the quality of the relationship between doctor and patient, developments over the past two decades have ensured that the physical components of the diagnosis and treatment, no less than the psychological and the social, have become subject to the same critical analysis. Although rarely described in these terms, Balint seminars and contemporary small group case discussions are among the most successful examples of medical audit in general practice in the United Kingdom. What may be missing is the recognition that these activities are a form of medical audit. They are, however, time consuming, their internal discipline is hard and takes time to learn, and the groups themselves need years rather than months to ensure that real learning and substantial change are taking place.

The audit of individual cases is likely to reveal two sources of error in the practice, knowledge of which can be invaluable. Firstly, *case specific* errors can be detected. The medication for a chronic condition may have been inappropriate, or incompatible drugs may have been used. It may be discovered that there has been no expert evaluation of the retina of a diabetic patient over a period of years. There may also have been *generic* errors, which point to the need to look at the organisation of the practice. Letters and reports may have been incorrectly filed; no action may have been taken on an abnormal laboratory finding, when this had been intended.

Finally, the audit of individual cases should not be confined to the sort of critical events described above. An important technique that was first developed in Balint groups, and much used now in case discussion groups, is that of *random case analysis*. If this is to be successful those engaged in the audit must commit themselves to sticking strictly to the rules of the engagement. The group may decide in advance the case to be discussed—for example, the third patient to be seen next Tuesday morning. It is of no account that the third patient on that Tuesday only wants to check something on a previously issued certificate, or is deaf and unable to communicate properly, or has arrived in the consulting room by mistake, intending to see the nurse. The doctor whose case has to be audited must commit himself to reporting that case and offer no excuse, however plausible, for choosing any other.

The ethos of medical audit

Modern general practice demands far more from the general practitioner than sound clinical practice. It demands the energetic management of a health service in miniature. With the advent of fund holding general practice, the scope of this management will become wider than previous experience has prepared us for, and the boundaries of the general practitioner's managerial responsibilities may eventually extend into many aspects of the specialist care of his or her patients in hospital.

Sound management, a prerequisite for the good quality of patient care, must be based on a clear vision of the intentions of the practice, an estimate of the size of, and the necessary resources for, the tasks to be undertaken, and a constant monitoring of performance against plans. The tools for this work, in essence the information and communication systems of the practice, are described on pages 196–223.

The concepts and techniques of medical audit are thus revealed as central to two linked tasks of general practice: solving clinical problems and managing the organisation. There is, however, a third task that medical audit must address and serve. General practice is not only a biotechnical enterprise and a managerial challenge; it is also a moral endeavour. The medicine of general practice is much concerned with optimising the resources of the individual, biological and psychological, spiritual and social, to cope with life's challenges and vicissitudes. It is concerned to represent the biotechnical possibilities of diagnosis and treatment on a human scale. It is concerned not with the fashionable—and perhaps fictional—battle between autonomy and dependency in the relationship between doctor and patient, but with a more subtle coming to an understanding with the patient about what he or she wants, needs, and is capable of achieving.

Part of this ethos is expressed in an appropriate openness between doctor and patient, and the new manifestation of this has been the growing interest in the accountability of the practice to the patients that it serves. The results of medical audit may thus in the future be reported not only to the practice personnel as a contribution to their professional development and the management of the practice but to the patients of the practice as a contribution to their own growing participation and personal responsibilities.

1 McIntyre N, Popper H. The critical attitude in medicine: the need for a new ethics. *Br Med J* 1983;**287**: 1919–23.
2 Berwick DM. Continuous improvement as an ideal in health care. *New England Journal of Medicine* 1989;**320**: 53–6.
3 Montagu A. Anthropology and medical education. *JAMA* 1963;**183**: 577.
4 McCormick J. Cervical smears: a questionable practice. *Lancet* 1989;ii: 207–9.
5 Donabedian A. *Exploration in quality assessment and monitoring*. Vol 1. Ann Arbor: Health Administration Press, 1980.
6 Irvine D. *Teaching practices*. London: Royal College of General Practitioners, 1972. (Report from general practice No 15.)
7 Burke P. Otitis media: is medical management an option? *J R Coll Gen Pract* 1989;**39**: 377–82.
8 Howie JGR, Porter AMD, Forbes JF. Quality and the use of time in general practice: widening the discussion. *Br Med J* 1989;**298**: 1008–10.
9 Hart JT. *Hypertension*. London and Edinburgh: Churchill Livingstone, 1980.
10 Balint M. *The doctor, his patient and the illness*. London: Tavistock, 1957.

Standards

MARSHALL MARINKER

Introduction

I began the previous chapter with a reference to science. This was in recognition of the fact that medical audit is nothing less than an attempt to apply scientific method to the quest for quality. Scientific method demands that the terms we use are clearly defined. For this reason science, wherever possible, is discussed and communicated in an invented language of clearly defined symbols. In real language the word "mercurial" carries associations with a god, a planet, a metal, and a medicine. The *Oxford English Dictionary* gives such meanings as eloquence, ingenuity, aptitude for commerce, volatility, sprightliness, and ready wit.

In the language of chemistry the symbol Hg signifies one thing and one thing only: it describes a silver-white metallic element with a specific atomic number and mass. To define a word for the purposes of scientific endeavour we have to diminish its meanings. This is true of the most commonly used term in the lexicon of medical audit and quality assurance. That word is "standard." In living language the word carries associations with a flag or pennant, a stick or post, and a tree. It carries such meanings as basic, average, unimaginative, usual, measured, uniform, conforming, traditional, authoritative, desired, and excellent.

For the purposes of this book I shall define a *standard* as the performance the auditors have set themselves to achieve. In much of the literature on audit the word is given a more limited and specific definition—to denote the quantity of a particular component of audit. This can be confusing, and here we shall use the term *target* for this more specific purpose.

Tracers

Before standards can be set decisions have to be taken about the aspects of the practice that are to be considered for standard setting. Medical audit cannot address every aspect of the practice's work, the whole range of clinical conditions, the whole age range, or every aspect of the practice's organisation. In the previous chapter reference was made to the principle of economy of effort. The aim of medical audit must be to achieve the greatest benefit in terms of improved patient care for the most modest expenditure of resources—time, money, and personnel. The chosen audit should therefore not only be capable of giving information about the particular aspect of care under scrutiny but, if possible, should throw light on more general aspects of the care given by each doctor, or by the practice as a whole. These subjects of medical audit, chosen for their ability to reveal many aspects of the practice's performance, are known as *tracer conditions*. To sample a whole range of practice activities it is necessary to create some sort of framework so that different tracers can be selected to reflect the practice as a whole.

Kessner et al[1] suggested using at least two tracer conditions that were relevant to both sexes and to four broad age groups, and that a useful tracer should meet the following criteria.

(1) A tracer should have a definite functional impact. By this I believe the authors mean that conditions that are not amenable to treatment, or that cause only negligible impairment, are unlikely to give useful information about the performance of the service being audited. A condition like pityriasis rosea, which is self limiting and for which there is no specific treatment, would make a poor tracer.

(2) A tracer should be well defined and easy to diagnose. Clearly hypertension would be well qualified. Depression, in contrast, because the diagnostic criteria are known to be much more elusive in general practice than they appear to be on the pages of psychiatric textbooks, might not qualify. If depression were chosen as a tracer a criterion such as the score on a well validated depression inventory rather than a diagnosis based solely on clinical judgment might be acceptable.

(3) The prevalence rate should be high enough to permit the collection of adequate data from the population sample. In general practice an audit of the management of all those patients with Crohn's disease would be inappropriate. The number of expected cases in a practice of average size would be too small. On the other hand, it would be perfectly possible to

carry out a confidential inquiry into the care of an individual patient with Crohn's disease.

(4) The natural history of the tracer condition should vary with the utilisation and effectiveness of medical care. Epilepsy and asthma would qualify well. Multiple sclerosis would not.

(5) The techniques of medical management of the condition should be well defined for at least one of the following: prevention, diagnosis, treatment, or rehabilitation. While this may be the easiest of Kessner's desiderata to satisfy, it should be remembered that Kessner requires all six of his desiderata if a tracer is to be regarded as really useful.

(6) The effect of non-medical factors on the tracer should be understood. In general practice there is a need to take heed of the socioeconomic environment in which the audit is being carried out. Socioeconomic factors have the most profound effect not only on the prevalence of many diseases but on such factors as the decision to seek help, the natural history of the disease, compliance with treatment, and, even in the National Health Service, the availability of health care resources. A failure to appreciate the impact of these factors on health and health care results in the creation of quite unrealistic expectations.

Performance indicators

The concept of performance indicators is closely related to that of tracers. The word "tracer" refers to the condition that is to be considered. The term "performance indicators" refers to the tasks which are carried out by the health care workers involved. Maxwell[2] argued that health services should be assessed in at least six dimensions: relevance to need, ease of access, effectiveness, fairness, social acceptability, and efficiency and cost. The creative management of general practices in the future will undoubtedly demand that attention be paid to all these six categories.

Best[3] identifies three criteria that validate a performance indicator. Firstly, the indicator must in some way be calibrated: "... this will usually mean that some measure of output will be expressed in relation to the input or inputs required to produce that output." Secondly, the indicator must be subject to unambiguous interpretation. Thirdly, changes in the indicator must be subject to influence by those whose performance is being judged. It would simply be dispiriting to identify need for change in a positive direction without either the authority or means to bring about such change.

Monitoring the practice's repeat prescription system would seem to fulfil all three of Best's criteria. Firstly, a system that controlled the quantities and frequencies of repeat prescriptions, permitted a review of duration and dosage, and checked for pharmacologically incompatible regimes would clearly have a direct relationship to "output." Secondly, the detection of inappropriate prescribing, or of failure of compliance with an important continuing medication, might be thought to be fairly unambiguous in interpretation. Thirdly, changes in the indicator would certainly be within the capacity and control of those whose performance was being assessed.

In contrast, the monitoring of rates of referral to hospital would not fulfil all these important criteria. Although movement in the indicator would certainly be subject to influence by the doctor whose performance is being judged, it would be quite impossible to calibrate the performance, still less to interpret movements towards more or fewer referrals as in any way indicating improvements or deteriorations in the quality of care. There is yet no research[4] that permits us to say that high, low, or mean rates of referral can be judged in terms of the appropriateness and quality of the doctor's referral practices.

The four chapters covering, respectively, chronic conditions, acute conditions, clinically significant events, and auditing practice management suggest a framework for selecting tracers. Clearly it is important that tracers be selected from at least each of the four major categories (or chapter headings) that we suggest. Which conditions are selected and how frequently there is a change of condition within each category are matters for practice policy. But practical considerations, the need to use limited resources for medical audit to best effect, suggest that practices should at any one time be economical in their choice of things to be audited.

Examples

As an example of the audit of patients with *chronic conditions* an audit of patients with diabetes mellitus will throw light on the practice's approach to the diagnosis, management, and monitoring of other chronic conditions. An audit of patients with schizophrenia will throw light on the management of psychiatric illness in a largely young adult population. An audit of palliative care will throw light not only on the practice's approach to the technical problems of therapeutics but also on the care of a more elderly population, on the approach to teamwork, and support for informal carers.

By the same token the choice of *acute conditions* to be monitored can also focus attention on particular age groups, or on particular aspects of the practice's performance. An audit of heart failure will focus on clinical and pharmacological skills in the care of older people. An audit of upper respiratory tract infection will focus on communication and health education skills in the care of young people and on the relationship between doctor, parent, and child.

The organisation of the practice can also be subjected to audit. Audits here might include the response of staff to medical emergencies; an audit of the record system and quality of the notes; an audit of the repeat prescription system; laboratory and imaging investigations; and referral letters to hospital consultants. All of this is predicated on the notion that criteria will be recognised, against which performance can be assessed.

An anatomy of standards

Having selected a tracer, the auditors next have to decide on a number of relevant *criteria* which can be measured. Criteria are components of the tracer condition that are thought to be relevant to the performance of the doctor or the practice. In the case of hypertension, for example, good criteria might include the percentage of discovered hypertensives in the adult population, the medications employed, and measurements of blood pressure after treatment.

A *standard* is created when these criteria are given certain quantitative or qualitative characteristics. Such standards in fact serve as *targets* and the reason for preferring this term is given at the beginning of this chapter. Our knowledge of the incidence of moderate to severe hypertension in an adult population, corrected for its age/sex structure, permits the practice to predict the approximate percentage of "cases " which could be found by total successful screening. The actual number of cases found after five years of opportunistic screening—that is, monitoring the blood pressure of all adults who present to the practice for no matter what clinical problem—can then be compared with this "expected" figure, so that some estimate can be made of the efficiency of the practice's screening programme. Other criteria may be used and targets may be agreed that will reflect other aspects of the care of hypertensive patients. What levels of blood pressure control were achieved? To what extent did the medication actually used comply with the range of drugs that the practice had agreed to employ?

A *protocol* for diagnosis or treatment is a statement about optimum performance. In the case of diagnosis the practice may wish to stipulate a number of necessary preconditions that must be met to establish the diagnosis. For example, in the case of hypertension the practice may demand that the blood pressure be taken on more than one occasion; it may specify whether the patient is sitting or standing; it may rely on measures of diastolic or systolic pressure, or both; it may decide on the highest readings, or the lowest readings, or the mean of all the readings. The literature on hypertension is unhelpfully replete with advice on this, much of it contradictory. Most general practices will resist the temptation to make a thorough search of the literature and a critical review of it. For the purposes of clinical audit there is often a consensus view that serves as a basis for standard setting. How is this consensus view formed?

Quite often this view begins with the opinions of specialists in a particular field, based on a mixture of their clinical experience and their interpretation of the literature. One of the major strengths of medical audit is that it compels the auditors to look with fresh eyes at received clinical wisdom. It is important to remember that for the most part textbook descriptions of disease, and textbook recommendations for treatment, are based on the experience of secondary medical care—on the experience of specialists who mostly see only those patients referred to them by general practitioners. The textbook picture is therefore both incomplete and potentially misleading. If standards are to be set for general practice they must be set in general practice. Some sort of dialogue will then be necessary not only between the general practitioners in partnership who wish to audit their own work but between general practitioners and the relevant specialists concerned. Such discussions and negotiations are described in the chapter on group work (pages 185–95).

Protocols may take many forms. They may consist of questions to be answered, of actions to be carried out, or of choices to be made. Sometimes a protocol is given the form of an *algorithm*, which is a graphic display of binary logic. These algorithms, if they are to reflect the wide range of possibilities and choices that are encountered in practice, can sometimes appear rambling and confusing. This is because the algorithm depicts not the way in which the doctor thinks but rather the way in which the computer has been taught to process. Clearly I dislike them.

Standards that are derived from textbook and specialist sources, even when mediated by general practice experience, are described as *ideal* or *normative*. The danger here is that these so called ideal standards may be unrealistic, and may sometimes be actually damaging. Standards can be unrealistic if they do not take into account the true prevalence and incidence of events in general practice. In past decades some of the protocols for optimum diagnosis and treatment in the United States begin to resemble the aggregated small print of major specialist textbooks written up as a brief for the defence in a law suit. Protocols in general practice should reflect the tasks of general practice. The task of the specialist[5] is to reduce uncertainty, to pursue possibility, and to marginalise error. The task of the general practitioner is to accept uncertainty, to explore probability, and to marginalise danger. General practice protocols should reflect general practice realities.

The general practitioner has to consider what uncertainties it is safe to tolerate when a child presents with acute pain in an ear obscured by wax; when he is consulted by a young woman who has unaccountably stumbled and fallen for a third time in a year; or when he considers what to do next for a middle aged woman whose indigestion persists despite alkali mixtures and cimetidine. What probabilities does he need to explore when an adolescent girl loses weight; when an octogenarian complains of giddiness on getting out of bed; when a young wife tells her doctor that her husband probably needs a good physical checkup? What dangers must be marginalised when a child presents with high fever; when a young woman presents with colicky abdominal pain; when an elderly widow comes to tell her doctor that her pet dog has had to be put down?

The clinical competencies of general practice are derived from values that have all but disappeared in late twentieth century medicine. What society values in our times is excellence in specialism: this demands a deep and penetrating understanding of a restricted field of endeavour, with an emphasis on technical skills, convergent thinking, rationality, and the explicit.

Excellence in generalism is quite different. It is characterised by a superficial grasp of a very wide field of endeavour; problem solving is horizontal rather than vertical; thinking is as much convergent as divergent; the skills are not so much technical as interactive; there is room not only for the rational and the explicit but also for the intuitive and the implicit.

The United Kingdom is both a multiracial and a multicultural society. Members of ethnic minorities exhibit particular patterns of morbidity, including morbidities that may be associated with the effects of immigration itself, and these may be manifest in the families of immigrants over more than one generation. Further, populations of ethnic minorities have their own particular social needs, health beliefs, expectations of medical care, and many other factors that can affect health, health care, and the way in which the practices that serve them can perform. Because of these factors, standard setting must be carried out with sensitivity to these important local variables. It is also worth recalling that even within the host or majority culture there may be local variables such as the socioeconomic structure of the practice population, the availability of health care resources, and so on.

When a protocol reflects these general practice realities the standards are described as *pragmatic*. The danger here is that the term, indeed the very idea, can be used as an alibi for poor or unacceptable standards. This does not have to be so. Pragmatic standards must above all be safe: that is to say they must fully explore probability and maximally marginalise danger.

Confidential inquiries

Perhaps the standards of care in which the doctor can have most trust are those that emerge from the search for avoidable errors in his or her own clinical work. I described this approach to the individual case in the preceding chapter. A group undertaking such a confidential inquiry into an individual significant event needs to pay attention to a number of issues in the quest for better standards. Six essential steps may be recalled by the use of the acronym REPOSE.

Firstly, the *reason* for the inquiry should be clearly stated. For example, a woman may have become pregnant while taking an oral contraceptive. It is discovered that she has also taken another prescribed medicine—an antibiotic which has possibly interfered with the contraceptive action of the pill. Next, the *evidence* needs to be presented. What evidence is there in the research literature of interaction between the pill and other medication? Partnerships will need to become confident in the critical reading of research evidence, not least in assessing the size of risk and the implications for clinical decision making in general practice. These considerations will result in the formulation of a *policy*. Experience, however, suggests that care must be taken to ensure that all those who will be involved in pursuing this policy understand it, agree with it, and are motivated to carry it out. This means that the audit group must ensure that those involved have a sense of *ownership* of this policy. When this has been done a *system* can be devised to ensure that the policy is adhered to—for example, the medical records of all women known to be taking oral contraceptives can, following consultation, be reviewed by the practice nurse to note compliance. Lastly, the audit group can agree to make *enquiry* at a given interval to ensure that compliance with the policy has been achieved. Only by attention to all these steps can the audit group repose trust in the validity of the standards that follow from such an exercise.

Norms

Finally, standards may be derived not from research or clinical opinion or local negotiation but rather from a belief in the inherent worth or statistical averages or *norms*. The longest established medical audit in British general practice, that of prescribing, is based on such a belief. Doctors are provided with statistics about their own prescribing, and are given as reference points the prescribing averages for their partnership, for their locality and region. These norms then become either implicit targets or, sometimes, implicit ceilings. No attempt is made to correlate the level of prescribing, in terms of the number of prescriptions issued or the average cost of prescriptions, with the quality of care. There is an undeclared consensus, or perhaps a conspiracy, to equate these norms with virtue.

The same would not be true if the Department of Health sought to apply such norms to judgments about rates of referral to hospital. In one major study[6] the difference in referral rates between doctors in the top and bottom quintiles of the study population was fourfold. Despite such large disparities, the researchers were unable to draw any conclusions linking rates of referral to the quality of care.

Judgments

Standards are sometimes referred to as *explicit* and *implicit*. Any standard which is to be applied to a population must be explicit—that is to say, it must be stated clearly and unambiguously, and wherever possible quantified. Difficulties arise, however, when we try to apply unambiguous explicit standards to individual cases—for example, in confidential inquiries or in sampling individual case notes where the audit reveals a departure from the standards set. Here judgments can only be made in relation to the clinical experience and values of the auditors. The auditors have to ask the questions: "What would we ourselves have done in these circumstances? What reasonable steps might have been taken? What external factors made it difficult or impossible to adhere to the agreed protocol?"

Sometimes it is possible to make explicit what might otherwise appear to be entirely implicit judgments. For example, the writer,[7] in judging the quality of case discussions, suggested the following catechism:

- Has the problem been effectively identified?
- Has the problem been resolved in the shortest possible time?
- Has the number of problem solving steps been reduced to a minimum consonant with safety?
- Has the simplest technology been employed?
- Has the optimum medication been selected and monitored?
- Has the management caused the minimum harm or risk of harm to the patient?
- Has there been optimum use of health care personnel?
- Have self care and family care been fully mobilised?
- What realistic criteria of success were adopted, and were they achieved?

One of the most commonly voiced objections to medical audit is that it is impossible to apply explicit standards (applicable to populations) to the individual case. This objection is valid, if such explicit standards are insensitively applied without recourse to implicit judgment. In judging an individual case explicit protocols should be used to pose questions about the clinical care. They must not be used simply to pass arbitrary judgments about what is good or bad.

Conclusion

The search for standards begins with some sensible and pragmatic questions about what we are trying to achieve. A group of doctors may begin with the question, "Why not look at how we treat depression?" They will be driven to ask, "How often do we make the diagnosis now, and what do we do about it?" Next they may ask, "How does my performance compare with that of others and is there anything that I can learn from this comparison?" Before too long, however, other questions suggest themselves: "What do we mean by the term depression?" and then "What is the received wisdom about this, and where is the evidence?"

Setting standards is the prerequisite of good management. Monitoring and achieving them are the goals of good management. But this alone is not enough. I began this chapter by considering the meanings that have attached themslves to the word. The word "standard" carries with it shades of authority, certainty, and permanence. But this is not the essence of clinical science. The search for standards demands a constant reconsideration of what we know, how we know it, and how we understand it. The search for standards is the purpose of medical audit. In this sense medical audit becomes the ultimate refresher course, in every meaning of that term.

1 Kessner DM, Kalk CE, Singer J. Assessing health quality—the case for tracers. *New England Journal of Medicine* 1977;**288**:189–94.
2 Maxwell RJ. Quality assessment in health. *Br Med J* 1984;**288**:1470–2.
3 Best GA. Performance indicators: a precautionary tale for unit managers. In: Wickings HI, ed. *Effective unit management*. King Edward's Hospital Fund for London, 1983:62–83.
4 Marinker M, Wilkin D, Metcalfe D. Referral to hospital: can we do better? *Br Med J* 1988;**297**:461–4
5 Marinker M. *Greening the White Paper*. London: Social Market Foundation, 1989.
6 Wilkin D, Smith AG. Variations in general practitioner's referral rates to consultants. *J R Col Gen Pract* 1987;**37**:350–3.
7 Marinker M. Case discussion. In: Cormack J, Marinker M, Morrell D, eds. *Teaching general practice*. London: Kluwer, 1981:105–11.

How to begin

MICHAEL DRURY, BILL STYLES

Even if you understand what audit is, and welcome its introduction, it is highly probable that some of your colleagues in the practice will be unclear about its purpose. Selling the idea to the whole practice and motivating each of its members are undoubtedly essential prerequisites. The word "audit," with its undertones of finance and being called to account, has the capacity to produce negative feelings in people who regard themselves as "giving" a service to patients in need. Yet it is likely that all those in the practice are already concerned with improving aspects of their work, and such improvement is the underlying purpose of medical audit. It can make important contributions to the further education and professional development of every member of the practice team, and it can make fundamental contributions to improving the quality of patient care. These are its essential benefits, and whatever arrangements are made for audit within a practice they must be directed towards these purposes. Although audit can be developed as an instrument of accountability, its main goals must relate to education and to standards of patient care.[1] Its success in these areas will depend upon the active participation of those practice members who together have agreed to review their own performance and the quality of their work.

It is likely that many members of the practice team have already been involved with audit procedures through simple projects undertaken within the practice, or by participating when visiting other practices, or through trainer selection procedures. The selection of general practitioner trainers on the basis of agreed regional criteria is one of the commonest exercises in medical audit in general practice. Nevertheless, the prospect of embarking upon medical audit in a more systematic and organised way will cause concern within every practice. These concerns will have to be addressed if future activities are not to be prejudiced by indifference or even by hostility within the practice team.

Possible obstacles and pitfalls

There will be a number of obstacles and pitfalls in the early stages. Therefore good groundwork at this point will prevent difficulties later on. Firstly, it is essential that everyone in the practice is briefed about the nature and the objectives of audit. Although it is possible to do this at a large practice meeting involving all staff, it is probably better to begin with a series of small meetings when the principles are still being debated. It is essential that the partners in the practice should be clear about the purpose of audit and committed to future activities involving it; so, too, must be all members of the practice staff. It is inevitable that some members of the group will be defensive, feeling that they do not have the necessary ability for work with audit. Others may have major reservations and misconceptions about what audit is and what purpose it serves. All these difficulties must be resolved early on, otherwise they will soon become the focus for discontent. People will be anxious about the time involved and will fear the intrusion of audit activities into what, for many, is already a busy working schedule. Some anxieties about time may reflect the doubts that members of the practice might have about their abilities to participate in such work and all this has to be explored in a sensitive way. Before long some will begin to show enthusiasm for the suggestion of being involved in audit projects and soon a series of proposals will begin to emerge. The next difficulty will be in considering everyone's different priorities so that a starting point can be determined.

At this stage it is worth reviewing once more the overall benefits of audit and why the practice is undertaking it. What does the practice team hope to learn from this work? How will it help each of the members in continuing education and professional development? How will it lead to more efficient practice management and to the more appropriate use of time and other practice resources? How will it contribute to more effective care and, in this way, benefit the patients in the practice? The practice must be clear from the start how the results of the audit exercise will be used.

Emphasis must be laid on the confidential nature of the work and the fact that it is designed to lead to improvements in the services of the practice through modification in practice routines and that most certainly it will not be linked to sanctions and to punishment of practice members. In the early stages most practices are content to limit the results of their audit activities to the members of the practice. As confidence and trust develop some are prepared to share their results and to compare them with other local practices, sometimes under the umbrella of local medical committees and of local faculties of the Royal College of General Practitioners.

Agreement within the practice team

Once the partners have agreed in general terms the purposes of the audit and how it will be undertaken, the broad concept should be discussed with the other members of the practice team and particularly with the practice manager, who will have a key role in designing and running systems that are introduced. The reservations and concerns that may already have been expressed and explored with the partners will undoubtedly be shared by the other members of the team. Once again, it is important to understand these fears and to ensure that each member of the practice understands the overall purpose of the audit exercises that are proposed.

Clinical audits on the care of specific conditions will almost certainly involve the nurses in the practice, whereas audits of the administrative procedures, such as appointment systems, hospital referrals, and so on, will be the concern of the practice receptionists and secretaries.

Sooner or later, for any audit, all practice staff will become involved so that it is important from the outset to have all members committed and convinced of the merit of the work that is proposed.

Everyone must be convinced of the value of the audit to them and their aspirations for patients. Early discussions will provide opportunities for practice staff to share their overall vision of the work of the practice. It will be important to focus on the area of work of each of them and to listen to their views. The cost of audit to them will have to be considered. Everyone will know at once that audit will take time and to people who already consider themselves busy this may seem to be yet another "last straw." A fear of lack of time will be a reasonable anxiety: it is often the excuse that some will use to hide from the threat that audit will expose deficiencies in their work. Such fears must be clearly understood by those proposing involvement in audit and the sensitive handling of such issues is vital if progress is to be made.

Most of us will have different agenda for this exercise and people will need to have an opportunity to put their priorities forward and to recognise that, as audit becomes a continuing programme, they will be able to organise their own activities. In any case, once each understands that audit is essentially educational he or she will soon realise that all of us learn from every audit. It is clearly important, however, that from the start subjects are chosen that are generally relevant to the care of patients and to the training of practice staff.

Time and enthusiasm are precious commodities that must not be squandered. The aims of audit tasks must therefore be realistic and the tasks should be capable of completion. Picking a subject for which it is too difficult to collect and analyse the data, or one for which it would be impossible to implement the necessary changes that it highlights, would be a bad start. It is much better to agree a relatively simple, albeit important and relevant objective, from which a result can be obtained before enthusiasm wanes. As people's confidence builds up it is possible to shift towards more esoteric and complex areas. It is much easier to bear failure at a later stage when successes have already been obtained; early failures can halt the programme.

What to audit

Having agreed to become involved in audit, the practice team must then decide on the activity to be studied. This can be an analysis of a clinical aspect of the practice's work or a review of one of the non-clinical systems that supports it. An example of the latter might be to review the efficiency of the practice's appointment system or the arrangements for access to out of hours care.

Having agreed the practice activity to be studied, the members of the practice team must then determine what they are trying to achieve in this particular area. The results of the audit will then indicate how successful the practice is in reaching its previously agreed targets. These results will form the basis upon which the practice will decide how to improve its performance in this particular area. A rerun of audit at a later date will then demonstrate how successful or otherwise the practice has been in bringing about the improvements the first audit had suggested were necessary.

In the language of medical audit (see pages 15–25) the practice will have decided the criteria for the audit activity—that is, the elements to be studied within the practice—as well as the standards that will operate. Standards are explicit statements that indicate precisely what the practice has agreed are the acceptable levels of performance for which it is aiming. Agreeing standards can be difficult: they should be realistic and achievable while being at a level the practice has yet to attain.

Type of audit: quantitative or qualitative?

Having decided the area of activity for audit, the practice must then agree how the audit will be undertaken. In general terms there are two types of audit. The first depends upon the collection and analysis of data about a large number of patients or events. The second does not have such a quantitative basis and is based on the review of the time leading up to a significant or critical event. Such an event might be the unexpected death of a patient, the emergency admission of an asthmatic child to hospital, a case of measles, a young woman with carcinoma of the cervix, or the onset of blindness in a diabetic patient. Such a qualitative audit would involve all members of the practice team associated with the patient and its success would depend considerably on the accuracy of practice records.

The more quantitative type of medical audit depends on meticulous forward planning—on agreeing the activity to be reviewed and the people who will be involved, together with the data that will be collected and analysed. There is a tendency to opt for activities that are easily measurable. Whereas this is certainly to be recommended for a practice that is becoming involved in audit for the first time, it must be recognised that easily measurable aspects of a practice's work are not necessarily the best measures of its overall quality of care. Easily measurable activities include a practice's preventive services—for example, the childhood immunisation rates or cervical cytology.

The review of the care of patients with chronic disease lends itself readily to quantitative medical audit. An essential early step is to agree a practice protocol for the care of the chronic disease being studied. Many practices have found the protocols for chronic conditions that have been prepared by the Royal College of General Practitioners to be good starting points for the generation of their practice's own standards and procedures. Other practice activities that are readily measurable include prescribing and the efficiency of the practice's appointment system.

Agreeing criteria and standards

Having determined the practice activity to be reviewed, the next step is to decide the objectives that the practice works towards. Criteria are those elements of care that will be counted or measured to determine the quality. The standards will represent the measurements that the practice has agreed will reflect an acceptable level of care. Value judgments are involved in determining both of these and they will reflect the views of individuals in the team, as well as the current objectives of the general medical care system, which will usually be based on the evidence of scientific research.

The question that the members of the practice must be able to answer at this early stage is: "What are we trying to achieve through this particular activity?" Linked to this will be concerns about a particular practice activity—clinical or organisational. They will then agree the purpose of the audit that they are embarking on. The next step will be to measure the practice's overall level of performance against the standards (objectives) that they have agreed, which are based on the views and evidence that they have collected. These will be linked to the aims of the practice for the activity being studied, particularly to the processes for achieving these aims and to the outcomes.

Standards can be generated in either of two ways: through a review of the medical literature on the subject and an analysis of the perceived wisdom at that time, *or* by collecting data about the practice's present level of performance and then agreeing future targets from the information that these will yield.

On some occasions the members of a practice may agree standards based on information obtained in both these ways.

The information generated from the research literature and from the practice itself will then form the basis for discussion so that agreed standards of care can be determined by all those involved in the audit exercise. These standards will then form the basis of the exercise itself.

Additional information is collected and can be obtained from the family health services authority or the health board (for example, about items of service activities) or from the Prescription Pricing Authority. Such information can be of great help in auditing certain practice activities. In general, however, the collection of data by the practice itself has much to commend it, since the information derived from it would be of greater accuracy than that obtained from sources outside the practice.

As experience with medical audit develops the practice members may wish to collect data not easily identifiable in the normal practice routine. The Birmingham Research Unit of the Royal College of General Practitioners has considerable experience in developing instruments for measuring practice activity analysis. It has produced a number of encounter sheets relating to consultation numbers and rates, home visits, prescriptions issued, and laboratory and x ray investigations. One of these, for referrals to specialists is reproduced on pages 33–6. Some practices have produced similar encounter sheets upon which details of consultations can be quickly recorded. These then form the basis for further analysis and comparison with the work undertaken in previous years or in neighbouring practices.

Comparing data

One of the exciting developments of medical audit is that it enables members of a practice to compare their level of activity and performance either with their own record in previous years or with the work undertaken in other practices. The faculties of the Royal College of General Practitioners provide opportunities for this to be done on a local basis, and the College's Birmingham Research Unit has acted as a focal point for the collection and analysis of data from practices throughout the country. Information can be fed back to the practices concerned, who can then compare their levels of performance with those of their peers.

Comparison of results from year to year, or between practices, is not possible with raw data. These have to be analysed further to permit such comparison. Thus we can list relatively easily the number of x ray investigations requested in a year, which may be important if we wish to make a simple statement about this fact. If, however, we wish to make meaningful comparisons between what we do now and what we did five years ago, or what we do and what the practice next door does, then we need to report our activities as *rates*. The number of x rays requested for every thousand patients

The Royal College of General Practitioners

PRACTICE ACTIVITY ANALYSIS

5. REFERRALS TO SPECIALISTS

This analysis is concerned with referrals made from general practice to specialists both operating within the N.H.S. The recording is continued over 4 weeks.

A seperate sheet is used by each participating doctor. When completed summarise the results in the appropriate places, complete the data return sheet and return the entire document to your group leader or directly to

P.A.A.
RCGP Research Unit
54 Lordswood Road
Birmingham B17 9DB

Page 2 contains the Instructions and Referrals Score Grid.
Page 3 contains the Consultations Table and special instructions
for simultaneous completion of Analysis 6, Visiting Profiles.
Page 4 contains the Data Return Sheet.

Page 2 INSTRUCTIONS   R E F E R R A L   S C O R E   G R I D

     A score is made each time a NEW REFERRAL is made. A new referral does not include one in which the further opinion of a specialist is sought for a patient who has already consulted him on a previous occasion with the same problem.
     The analysis is only concerned with patients seen by the general practitioner under the N.H.S. and referred to specialists under the provisions of the N.H.S.

	O. P. OUT PATIENTS CLINIC	D. C. DOMICILIARY CONSn.	H. A. HOSPITAL ADMISSION
Dermatology	1 2 3 4 5 6 7 8 9 10	1 2 3 4 5	1 2 3 4 5
E. N. T.	1 2 3 4 5 6 7 8 9 10	1 2 3 4 5	1 2 3 4 5
Geriatrics	1 2 3 4 5 6 7 8 9 10	1 2 3 4 5	1 2 3 4 5
Gynaecology	1 2 3 4 5 6 7 8 9 10	1 2 3 4 5	1 2 3 4 5
Medicine	1 2 3 4 5 6 7 8 9 10	1 2 3 4 5	1 2 3 4 5
Obstetrics	1 2 3 4 5 6 7 8 9 10	1 2 3 4 5	1 2 3 4 5
Ophthalmology	1 2 3 4 5 6 7 8 9 19	1 2 3 4 5	1 2 3 4 5
Orthopaedics inc. Trauma	1 2 3 4 5 6 7 8 9 10	1 2 3 4 5	1 2 3 4 5
Paediatrics	1 2 3 4 5 6 7 8 9 10	1 2 3 4 5	1 2 3 4 5
Psychiatry	1 2 3 4 5 6 7 8 9 10	1 2 3 4 5	1 2 3 4 5
Surgery	1 2 3 4 5 6 7 8 9 10	1 2 3 4 5	1 2 3 4 5
Other	1 2 3 4 5 6 7 8 9 10	1 2 3 4 5	1 2 3 4 5

SUMMARISE RESULTS

	O. P.	D. C.	H. A.
Dermatology			
E. N. T.			
Geriatrics			
Gynaecology			
Medicine			
Obstetrics			
Ophthalmology			
Orthopaedics inc. Trauma			
Paediatrics			
Psychiatry			
Surgery			
Other			

CONSULTATIONS TABLE

Keep a record of all patients consulting during the FOUR study weeks and enter in the table. (Consultations for private patients are not included.)

WEEK 1					WEEK 2			
CONSULTATIONS a.m.	p.m.	VISITS	CLINICS		CONSULTATIONS a.m.	p.m.	VISITS	CLINICS
				MON				
				TUE				
				WED				
				THUR				
				FRI				
				SAT/SUN				

WEEK 3					WEEK 4			
				MON				
				TUE				
				WED				
				THUR				
				FRI				
				SAT/SUN				

CONSULTATIONS TOTAL   AM .... PM .... VISITS .... CLINICS...............

GRAND TOTAL ....

REFERRALS & VISITING PROFILES

These two analyses (5 & 6) can be undertaken simultaneously. In such cases the following procedure is recommended.

The recording doctor keeps the REFERRALS analysis scoring appropriately as and when referrals are made during the four study weeks. The consultations table (above) should be completed by him obtaining necessary information from the reception staff.

'VISITING PROFILES' should be given to the reception staff and scored for any 2 of the 4 weeks during which referrals are recorded. Scoring can be made either from the patients stated age or recorded date of birth. Visits made by the doctor must be reported to the receptionist by the doctor or scored personally by him. The procedure for scoring visits made by deputies, detailed in the Instructions for Visiting Profiles, should be explained to the receptionist.

DATA RETURN SHEET

To obtain a personal and group analysis of your recorded data complete this sheet and return to the leader of your recording group or directly to the Research Unit. (Address on Page 1)

Dr. Name . . . .

Partnership . . . .

Address . . . .

. . . .

Is this the first P.A.A. Data Sheet you have returned to the P.A.A. Unit.

YES ☐   NO ☐

Recording Group (if any) . . . .

Study Period From . . . . to . . . . (enter dates)

Type of Practice (enter one √ on each line)

1	Industrial ☐	Residential ☐	Mixed ☐
2	Urban ☐	Rural ☐	Mixed ☐
3	Dispensing ☐	Non-Dispensing ☐	Mixed ☐

Status of Recorder

Partner ☐   Assistant ☐   Trainee ☐

Practice List Size

Specify Total List Size . . . .

* Estimated Personal Contribution to Practice

During Study Period . . . . %

* Examples

Three partners sharing work load equally
Estimated Contribution = 33%

Four partner practice. One on holiday during study and of remaining three one worked part time.
Estimated Contribution = 40%

Single handed doctor. Occasional help with surgeries.
Estimated Contribution = 90%

Trainee. Not possible to estimate.
Estimated Contribution = N.K.

registered, or the number of *x* rays for every thousand consultations, provides information that can be much more readily compared. Another example would be the number of prescriptions issued for antihypertensive drugs. These might be declared as a rate for every thousand patients seen or, more meaningfully, as a rate for every hundred hypertensive patients seen.

Rates are expressed as so many items for so many people or events. The number of items counted, which is the number on top of a ratio, is known as the *numerator*. The number at the bottom of the ratio is the *denominator*; it refers to the population in which the event was studied. Rates are much more important markers of activity than crude numbers. Generally all numerical data generated in audit should be declared as rates if they are to allow further analysis and if comparisons are to be meaningful. Within the practice there are a variety of denominators that can be used, and the practice's age/sex register and morbidity index will be helpful in constructing these.

Age/sex register

Although some family practitioner committees will provide age/ sex registers free of charge, they are still maintained by only a minority of practices and only used by a proportion of the practices that have them. They have been thought by some doctors to be research tools. Although they are a key feature for research in general practice, they can contribute much to the efficient management of the practice and will be essential if the practice wishes to develop a full range of medical audit exercises; for example, it is not possible to know which 12 year old girls in the practice are immunised against rubella unless the practice has a list that distinguishes that practice population by age and sex. This will be important for any practice that needs to know the proportion of preventive services it undertakes and if it wishes to maximise or check its income.

Until recently many practices have kept an age/sex register by means of a card index system listing males and females in groups by year of birth. These cards have been marked or tagged to indicate, say, which of the patients have had their blood pressure recorded within five years and which, more importantly, have not. It is immediately apparent how such a simple system can be used in audit. If, for example, the practice agrees that all patients between the ages of, say, 30 and 65 should have their blood pressure recorded every five years then it is possible by using a tagged age/sex card system to know for how many this has been achieved and how many will need to have their blood pressures measured to secure a 100% target. To undertake such a simple audit exercise would be almost impossible without a tagged age/sex register.

The development of computers within general practice makes it much easier to develop an age/sex register and to keep it up to date. The importance of updating the practice age/sex register should be emphasised; it must be as accurate as possible since it provides one of the most important denominator populations for medical audit in general practice, namely the registered patient list. There is much to be said for practice staff ensuring every quarter that the practice age/sex register is up to date by checking that all new patients who have registered in the previous three months are included in the register and that those who have left have had their names removed from it. There is also a considerable advantage in comparing at regular intervals the age/sex register held in the practice with that held by the family practitioner committee or health board.

There are many other uses for the age/sex register, particularly for simple practice management as a directory of names, addresses, and telephone numbers, and as a profile of the practice for planning purposes, especially when it includes details of social class and ethnic groups.

The morbidity index

The second source of denominators within a practice population is the morbidity index. This provides lists of the patients who have particular problems that interest the practice. A few hundred practices, and particularly those involved in the national morbidity survey and the weekly return services of the Royal College of General Practitioners, have developed complete morbidity recording. Every diagnosis made in these practices is classified according to a coded system and is listed under the appropriate heading. This enables the practice or researchers working with it to determine how many new diagnoses of a particular condition are made each year (the incidence of the problem) and how many patients are on the list suffering from that problem (the prevalence of the problem). For example, a practice of 10 000 people may have 700 patients with asthma: so that the prevalence of asthma is 7%. Within the year only 20 new diagnoses of asthma may have been made, giving an incidence of 0.2%.

For most practices a more limited form of morbidity index will be appropriate. It will be for each practice to decide upon the medical conditions and special interests that it wishes included in its own index; for example, practices whose members wish to organise special sessions for the care of patients with asthma, diabetes, or hypertension will need accurate lists of all patients with these conditions so that they can monitor certain aspects of their care. Thus the morbidity index will be the starting point for determining the denominator population for audit of the quality of care of these patients.

Once the criteria for their care have been agreed, the patients with the condition being studied can be identified from the morbidity index and the medical records of each can then be reviewed to determine the extent to which the agreed standards for care have been applied. For example, are they being followed up at appropriate intervals? Is the information that was agreed to be essential being recorded properly? Is the control achieved, for example, of blood pressure levels and of blood sugar levels, measuring up to the agreed standards for good care?

Such data, acquired from the patient's individual medical record, is needed to monitor management against the practice's agreed standards. So, too, is a morbidity index to provide the denominator population.

The use of the computer in medical audit

Age/sex registers and morbidity indexes have been developed in practices for many years and, necessarily, have been kept in a manual way. The advent of the computer in general practice is rapidly changing this and makes the use of these registers and indexes much easier and quicker. The age/sex register of the practice must be included in any general practice computer program and this is so for most of the commonly used systems in general practice at the moment. Computers can print out lists and sublists of categories of patients and in this way they can contribute considerably to audit.

Most systems can produce the names and addresses of all

children and different age groups and so allow the measuring, for example, of the proportion of children who have not been immunised and for whom special measures will need to be taken. Such information is essential for the proper management of the practice and for maximising its income. It also enables the practice to measure how close it is to achieving its agreed targets for immunisation performance, and in the light of this to plan how to improve its procedures and to work toward higher standards of preventive care for the children in the practice population. The next stage is to repeat the audit cycle by measuring the effect of the changes that have been made earlier to ensure that they have resulted in the improvements that were considered necessary.

As the practice moves to a more sophisticated system, with a computer terminal in every consulting room and a diagnosis recorded on computer at every consultation, a computer held morbidity index will be built up and its use as an instrument to audit disease categories will be further enhanced.

The prescribing of new or repeat prescriptions through the computer also enables it to provide information about further subgroups within the practice population and thereby provide a different range of denominators; for example, the number of women on the contraceptive pill, the number of men on antihypertensive drugs, and those on anticonvulsant or antiasthmatic medication are denominators of population that can provide the basis for further audit studies.

Qualitative audit

Most of the audit work that has been undertaken to date in general practice has been of a quantitative type. Many practices have enjoyed collecting and analysing information about subgroups of patients within the practice population. The computer is making such work easier and has added an impetus to this type of activity. Qualitative audit is not based on the analysis of numbers or on large subgroups of a practice population. Nevertheless, some find it more challenging intellectually than quantitative audit, for it gets closer to the caring aspect of practice and to examining the extent to which each patient's real needs are met. Through qualitative audit the social and psychological components of care can be more easily examined. Nevertheless, qualitative audit can be as rigorous as quantitative audit, provided that the criteria agreed have been carefully defined.

In essence, qualitative audit consists of reviewing the records of patients and analysing on an individual basis whether or not the quality of care has met the standards that have been agreed by the practice. An analysis of this kind is usually triggered by a significant or critical event, and practices should agree in advance the events that might lead to such a review of patient care. Hospital obstetricians have undertaken such work for many years through the review of perinatal deaths, a review that most obstetric units carry out on a regular basis.

In the obstetric system of audit every case is rigorously examined by the group of doctors involved, to see that everything that had been agreed previously has been done. Were all the tests that should have been carried out in the prenatal period done? Was the labour managed appropriately? Were the grieving relatives treated properly? Was the general practitioner informed quickly? Given enough cases, this work can be quantified, but its value lies in the careful review of each case so that action for improvement can be taken on the basis of one single review.

In general practice there is a series of events that can be reviewed in this way. Although some of these might include the death of patients, and particularly their sudden death, they may not all be based on such an outcome; for example, the emergency admission of a child with asthma to hospital could provide a worthwhile basis for the exercise. Others might include a young woman with diagnosed cervical cancer, or a request for termination of pregnancy, or a relapsed schizophrenic patient. The list is endless and careful selection is needed to ensure that the topic being audited is important, relevant, and capable of giving a reasonably quick answer that can lead to improvement.

Collaborative audit

As competence with medical audit grows within a practice its members will wish to share their experiences and compare their results with others. In some localities medical audit groups have been established in postgraduate medical centres and in some instances through the local faculty of the Royal College of General Practitioners. In these groups some presentations are made of audits undertaken in particular practices, but mostly general exercises are developed so that the same aspects of care can be compared between practices. On some occasions special data collection forms have been agreed so that comparisons can be made. Many have found this work stimulating and enjoyable and a potent way of encouraging progress. The importance of ensuring that the data can be analysed in a manner that permits comparisons between practices cannot be overstated. In particular, the denominator population between the practices must be the same and results must be expressed as comparable rates.

Audit at the interface between hospital and general practice

As audit techniques develop there will be opportunities for collaborative audit between those working in general practice and those in the hospital setting. There will be occasions when activities at the interface itself can be monitored—for example, the appropriateness of hospital referrals; the delay in outpatient appointments; the communication between general practitioners and hospital specialists; and the efficiency of procedures before discharge from hospital, particularly for the elderly. There will also be opportunities to review together the care of patients with selected groups of chronic conditions and to compare the utilisation rates of laboratory and x ray facilities between hospital and general practice based colleagues.

Tracer conditions

It is not possible to audit every aspect of general practice or every medical condition seen within that setting. Some are easier to study than others, and these usually form the basis for tracer conditions. The assumption is made that the quality of care demonstrated for certain tracer conditions is a reasonably accurate measure of the quality provided for all the other illnesses dealt with in general practice.

The characteristics of a tracer condition are as follows:
- It should have a definite functional impact on those affected
- The condition should be well defined and easy to diagnose
- Its prevalence rate should be high in order to provide adequate numbers for study

- Its natural history must be modified by suitable treatment
- Its management must be well defined in terms of prevention, diagnosis, treatment, or rehabilitation
- The effect of non-medical factors on the tracer condition should be understood.

Using these criteria many tracer conditions can be identified in general practice. These would include chronic conditions such as hypertension, diabetes mellitus, epilepsy, asthma, and thyroid disease, as well as more acute disorders such as otitis media and urinary tract infection. A practice's morbidity index, particularly if computerised, will readily provide populations of these patients for medical audit purposes.

Using the results of medical audit

It should be agreed at the outset who is responsible for analysing the data and preparing the results. It is essential that the results should be presented in writing to all those members of the practice team who have been involved in the exercise. There should be an opportunity at a suitable meeting for all involved to come together to consider the results and how they will be used.

Consideration should be given to the audit exercise itself. How effective has it been? Was the experience as unpleasant as some had thought it might be? How could it have been improved? Were the data that were collected appropriate and might there have been better ways of gathering the information? Were the standards that were agreed reasonable ones? Was the project overall well designed and relevant to the needs of the practice?

Then the results of the exercise must be considered. What lessons can be learnt from them? How much more effort is needed for the practice to reach its agreed standards? Who will be responsible for bringing about some of the changes that have been found to be necessary?

By the end of the audit exercise there should emerge a management plan for the future. This should identify clearly the people who will be responsible for its implementation so that the results of the project can be directed towards better quality patient care.

The audit cycle

The members of the practice must also consider when they will next repeat an audit in this particular area of practice activity.

Then, on that occasion, the details for the next round of the audit cycle must be agreed and must take account of the many lessons learnt from the previous effort. In this way the effects of implementing the changes found by previous audit exercises can be measured and the overall success of the audit itself can be demonstrated for that particular activity. To undertake a single audit exercise within a given practice activity is fruitless. The strength of audit is its cyclical nature and the opportunity that it provides for measuring the effects of changes in practice routine that have been stimulated by previous audit procedures. Michael Sheldon[2] has demonstrated the five steps of medical audit, emphasising the importance of step 5, which is to repeat the audit exercise to find out whether or not the care of patients has improved as a result of previous efforts. Only by doing this can audit itself be audited.

Guidance and some warnings

It may help at this point to sum up the factors for success in medical audit. These are as follows:

- Agreement on the value of audit
- Agreement on the purpose of audit
- Taking account of the concerns of partners and practice staff (suspicion, lack of time, perceived lack of skills)
- Agreement on the practice activities to be studied
- Agreement on roles, especially for data collection, analysis, and reporting results
- Agreement on standards, based on a review of the literature and/ or present levels of practice activity
- Ensuring that the area of study is relevant
- Ensuring that data collection is easy, based on data already available within the practice
- Ensuring that the denominator population is well defined
- Ensuring that the condition studied is common in general practice
- Ensuring that the results can lead to the implementation of change
- Ensuring that the results are clearly expressed
- Ensuring that the results are considered
- Identifying those responsible for implementing the changes agreed to be necessary

- Agreement on a date for the rerun of an audit
- Completion of the audit cycle.

It may also help to give warnings about the problem areas to look for. These include the following:

- Information gathering in itself does not constitute audit: analysis is needed
- Agreement on standards is not easy and can cause difficulties
- Data collection can be laborious, particularly if it is not perceived as relevant and if it is not part of the normal practice routine
- Securing the involvement of all members of the practice
- Poor and impractical design of a project that requires excessive servicing will lead to problems
- The lack of a clear purpose for a project causes problems
- Poor practice records and no clear denominator population will cause failure.

Conclusion

Medical audit will soon become an everyday practice activity. It is important to ensure that the time and effort spent produces good results, so that the practice can be managed more efficiently and so that the quality of care available to patients can be enhanced. Once overcome, the suspicion and resistance to audit shown by some doctors and practice staff will give way to enjoyment and enthusiasm as the relevance of audit work to the work of the practice becomes apparent. Its success will depend upon maintaining the confidentiality of those involved and on dealing sensitively with any concerns that are expressed by practice staff. Audit must never be seen as a punitive exercise, with punishment and sanctions. It must be developed as an important part of the quest for higher standards of patient care. The elements for success include practice records of high quality, age/sex registers and morbidity indexes, as well as time when members of the practice can meet together to discuss this aspect of their work, to plan it carefully, to consider the results achieved, and to agree the changes in practice routine that may be found necessary.

1 Pendleton D, Schofield T, Marinker M. *In pursuit of quality—approaches to performance review in general practice.* London: Royal College of General Practi-

tioners, 1986; Baker R. *Practice assessment and quality of care.* London: Royal College of General Practitioners, 1988. (Occasional paper 39.); and Watkins CJ. *The measurement of quality in general practitioner care.* London: Royal College of General Practitioners, 1981. (Occasional paper 15.)

2 Sheldon G. *Medical audit in general practice.* London: Royal College of General Practitioners, 1982. (Occasional paper 20.) (Butterworth Prize Essay 1981.)

Where to begin

IAN BOGLE

Introduction

There is one overriding consideration before selecting a project for medical audit and that is that there should be a probability that the quality of care will be improved with consequent benefit to patients. Whatever motives others may have in initiating audit exercises, such as the management of resources or the containment of costs, for doctors the overall objective of improving the service to those in their care must be paramount.

In its white paper *Working for Patients*[1] the government recognises the value of medical audit in both the hospital and the contractor services. While it recognises the initiatives that are already taking place in practices it expresses the intention to work with the medical profession nationally to establish a system of medical audit in general practice. The working paper *Medical Audit* sets out the further thinking by the government on this subject.[2] It commits itself to certain fundamental principles that include the participation of every doctor in a medically led system of audit that has been agreed locally between the profession and the family practitioner committee. The obvious differences between the approach to medical audit in the hospital and primary care services are emphasised.

The contractual changes for general practitioners that took place from 1 April 1990 highlight certain areas where the doctor should begin audit activity either to ensure compliance with the terms of service or to maximise the income generated from the practice. In most of these studies, such as those that examine immunisation and vaccination rates, there can be substantial benefits in improved patient care, but the doctor will also benefit in increased job satisfaction and should not feel at all apologetic for using medical audit to improve the income of the practice. Increasing the amount of money earned for services given to patients is not something of which we should be ashamed.

There are certain basic considerations that must be discussed by partners in a practice before beginning even the simplest study. These can be identified under the following headings.

Partner agreement

Audit within a practice will not be successful unless it has the support of all the partners. The subject and methods should be agreed, as should the ways in which the resulting information is to be used. Audit of professional activities can be perceived as extremely threatening by the partners, but if the correct ground work is done within the practice this feeling can be minimised.

Financial implications

Any exercise in audit will have financial implications. These may be small—for example, the purchase of notebooks and a calculator—or they may be more significant, involving computers, computer software, extra staffing, etc. Whatever the financial consequences are they should be considered and agreed by the partners before the project starts.

Staffing levels

Continuing appraisal of practice activity will mean additional staff time. The partners should identify not only what extra time is likely to be required but also the members of staff who will be involved. These could include the receptionist, the secretary, or the practice nurse. It might even be necessary to take on another partner.

Record keeping

It has long been recognised that one of the foundations of efficient and good quality medical practice is the keeping of concise, accurate, and clear records. The records in the practice must be of a high standard before medical audit can be done successfully.

Partners should agree a minimum standard for the records,

which should at least mean having them in date order, with summary cards of main events attached. Data cannot be retrieved if a basic standard is not adhered to by all members of the practice team, including any temporary members such as trainee practitioners or locum doctors.

The practice list

Having decided upon certain practice standards for the patients' records, it is then important to check that the medical records held by the practice are not at variance with the family practitioner committee's list of patients registered with the practice. It is absolutely vital that the population identified by the practice and the family practitioner committee are the same, particularly when some payments to the practice are based on the achievement by the practice of certain targets. Unfortunately there is no way to check the practice population, other than to obtain a list of patients from the family practitioner committee and check the medical record cards held by the practice against it.

Subjects for audit

The partners should, at this stage, identify what information will be needed from the medical record cards. This may be extremely varied—for example, immunisation status, date of last cervical smear, blood pressure reading, or identification of certain diseases, such as diabetes. If it is not decided at the beginning of the exercise which subjects are to be studied the practice will be involved in a repetitive trawl through the patients' records that will not only be time consuming but will lead the practice staff to the conclusion that audit is a boring and fairly non-productive exercise.

The previous paragraphs have identified the basic problems that must be solved before starting to audit any practice activity. The next step is to consider the subjects to be audited, and it would seem sensible to start by looking at the changes brought about by the 1990 general practitioners' contract.

The introduction of target payments and differential night visit fees make it financially prudent that a practice has clear knowledge of these activities, since payment is made on information that the practice itself will have to provide, rather than relying on figures produced by the family practitioner committee or health authority. Similarly the introduction of certain obligations under the terms of service in relation to prescribing, services to elderly patients, and the monitoring of hospital referrals make it essential that these matters are the subject of audit within the practice.

It would therefore seem that these six subjects make very appropriate starting points for practice audit, as well as being of significant benefit to the practice in terms of income generation.

Immunisation and vaccination

The study of immunisation levels in a practice population is an excellent starting point for audit activity. It is the perfect example of a service given by a practice which has proven and unarguable benefit to patients. It also has the advantage that once gaps in provision have been identified it is possible to take some action to improve performance.

In the white paper *Promoting Better Health*[3] the government first refers to the consideration of incentives that might be incorporated in the remuneration system to achieve specified target levels for the provision of immunisation and vaccination. This was introduced into the 1990 contract against the advice of the medical profession and consequently amendments were made to the statement of fees and allowances. For calculation for target purposes, the immunisations have been divided into three groups:

Group 1 (three doses)	Group 2 (three doses)	Group 3 (one dose)
diphtheria	pertussis	measles
tetanus		mumps
poliomyelitis		rubella

Two target levels have been introduced—70% and 90%—and payment is calculated on the cover achieved by a general practitioner taking the average of the three groups. The target population is the number of 2 year old children on the doctor's medical list. The level of remuneration will be decided by which target is reached and by the proportion of immunising final doses performed by practitioners, as part of general medical service. It can therefore be seen that a practice will need to identify the 2 year old patients on the list at any particular time, the immunisation status of these children, and the place where the immunisation was done.

As this subject is a good example of a relatively simple audit process the detailed steps in the following paragraphs can be applied to setting up studies of other subjects. Most of the work can be done by properly briefed ancillary staff.

Identifying the target population

A practitioner with a list size of 2000 patients will have, on average, 22 patients who are 2 years old. The names and addresses of these patients will need to be verified with the family practitioner committee list of registered patients, so that the target population can be agreed.

Immunisation status

Reference to the patient's medical record should show which of the seven doses in the three different groups have been given. There will, however, probably be a small number of patients whose immunisation status is not known, or where for some reason the procedure has not been carried out at all.

Place of immunisation

Immunisation will have been performed either at a general practitioner's surgery or at a health authority clinic. The place of immunisation should be obvious from the records, but there may be some patients in whose records it has not been made clear.

Further investigation

If there are gaps in the information about whether a child has been immunised or where a procedure has taken place the patient will need to be followed up. The parents should be contacted by the practice, either through the health visitor or practice nurse, and the full picture of the immunisation state in the practice population should be completed.

Continuous updating

As well as setting up the system for patients already on the practice list, a means of identifying the immunisation status of all new patients will need to be introduced. This will include some patients who have been partially immunised elsewhere. The names of new babies must be recorded so that appropriate immunisation can be offered according to the agreed schedule.

The audit procedure for immunisation and vaccination should be set up by the ancillary staff. The performance of the practice in relation to preschool booster injections should be tackled in the same way, and at the same time. The information can be entered on a card filing system, either allied to, or separate from, the age/sex register. If the practice is computerised the information will be stored in the practice computer.

The advantage of this audit procedure is that it identifies immunisation deficiencies in the practice population, thereby enabling the partners to correct these by a special programme of immunisation, either at the surgery or, if necessary, at the patient's home. It can be carried out quite easily by ancillary and attached staff and it puts the partners in a position to be able to calculate the income due to them from target payments.

This is a two stage exercise as practitioners will need to ascertain whether they have achieved the 70% or 90% target figure and then proceed to calculate the income from their knowledge of the percentage of completing injections that have been carried out in general practice.

From a financial point of view, this audit exercise must be continuous as claims for payment will need to be made every quarter. Therefore the importance of keeping the system simple and up to date cannot be overstressed. It may well be that the registration interview with new patients to the practice will provide the opportunity to gather useful information.

Cervical cytology

What you have to do to introduce audit of cervical cytology in your practice has much in common with what you do for immunisation levels. *Promoting Better Health*[3] sets out the government's belief in the value of cytology screening in the early detection of cervical cancer, a view that is shared by the medical profession. It therefore conforms with one of the basic requirements of a subject to be audited: that it can be shown to bring benefit to patients.

It also is a subject of further interest to general practitioners in that it is the second instance in the 1990 contract (immunisation being the first) where item of service payments have been replaced by target payments. The target population in this case consists of all women between the ages of 25 and 64. The targets to be achieved are 50% for a lower level payment and 80% for a higher one. Patients who have undergone hysterectomy can be excluded from the target population. As the onus is on the doctor to make and substantiate a claim it will obviously be necessary for all general practitioners to know the "cytology status" of women on their list. The level of remuneration will finally be decided by which target is reached and by the proportion of tests carried out by the practitioner.

There is therefore a great similarity between the steps that must be gone through to set up a process for auditing cervical cytology and those for studying immunisation levels.

Identifying the target population

The names and addresses of all women aged 25 to 64 will have to be compared with a list obtained from the family practitioner committee and any anomalies will have to be sorted out. It will be a much more time consuming task than that involving the 2 year old population for immunisation screening, owing to the greater number of patients involved. This part of the exercise, however, should be carried out by the practice ancillary staff.

Cervical cytology status

In this sensitive area patients would expect the results to remain confidential. In many practices it would be wise for the doctor to verify the results of the tests. It may be that statistics from health authority records will be satisfactory for the practice, but deriving data directly from the medical record card is usually a much more accurate method, especially with regard to the identification of patients who have had a hysterectomy.

Place of smear testing

The medical record card will show where a smear test was done. It may have been at a general practitioner surgery, at a health authority clinic, or at a special session arranged, for example, by a major commercial company. The place where a smear test is done should be recorded, if it is known.

Further investigation

It is assumed for the sake of this example that the practice is following the five year recall pattern referred to in the 1990 contract and which is the basis of the target remuneration system.

It is easily adapted to fit other recall cycles, such as every three years. From a search through the patients' medical record cards, various groups will have been identified.

Smear tests within the last five years—These patients' details should be recorded in a card filing system, or on computer, and placed in the order in which the patients will need to be recalled—that is, patients screened five years ago at the front and those most recently screened at the back.

Hysterectomy performed—These patients should be excluded from the target population as far as calculation for remunerative purposes is concerned. It may well be that in some cases the doctor will decide that a vault smear is indicated on clinical grounds.

Smear test outside the last five years—Unless there are compelling reasons for not doing so these patients should be sent for and offered an appointment to attend the cervical cytology clinic at the practice. If patients fail to attend the clinic and do not indicate that they do not wish the test to be done it may be appropriate for the practice nurse to follow them up at home. This will require handling with delicacy and diplomacy.

No knowledge of smear tests—Normally, these patients should be contacted and offered an appointment to attend the clinic. Subsequent action would be as indicated above.

Smear test not wanted—In a few medical record cards it may be indicated that the patient does not wish a test to be carried out. These patients should be identified so that they are not bombarded with constant reminders to attend unless the doctor decides that changed circumstances make it appropriate for the patient to be approached again.

Continuous updating

A system for identifying the cytology status of patients new to the practice and who are in the target age group will need to be devised. It is also wise to record information about cervical smears performed on patients in a younger age range, so that they can be incorporated easily into the system at a later date.

Much of the work of setting up an audit system for cervical cytology can be done by ancillary staff, although medical input will also be needed. Once a practice has set up a system it can be easily updated so as to keep a continuous record of practice performance. It not only puts in place a highly satisfying audit system but it also produces benefits that are clear to the patients while allowing the practice to maximise its income from this activity.

It must be emphasised that this description has been concerned with the use of the cervical smear test as a screening device and not as a diagnostic test. When, however, a diagnostic test is carried out on a patient the results of such a test must be fed into the practice system.

PACT

In *Promoting Better Health* the government stresses the importance of the prescribing information system that has been developed with the full cooperation of the medical profession.[3] Audit of prescribing in general practice, using information from this system, was referred to in the 1990 contract, where a change in the terms of service for general medical practitioners requires them to submit an annual report containing information about "practice policies for effective and economic prescribing." In addition, *Working for Patients* introduced the concept of indicative prescribing budgets and practice budgets that, to make the schemes operate efficiently, would require improved information systems.[1]

For these very practical reasons, it is clear that a practice must monitor its prescribing patterns. The advantages of making this one of the first subjects for audit is that the information is available, is collected efficiently by an agency outside the practice, and is sent to all general practitioners at regular intervals. Audit of prescribing will bring benefit to patients if the information gained from it is used to make changes that give maximum therapeutic benefit in the most cost effective way.

PACT stands for "prescribing analyses and cost," and PACT information is produced at three levels. Level 1 provides basic information in terms of practice prescribing costs, the number of items dispensed, and their average cost (figure 1). It also highlights the practice's prescribing patterns in six major therapeutic groups in terms of the number of items dispensed and the total cost. Finally, it gives the basic information about the prescribing habits of each doctor within the practice framework, and indicates the percentage of items prescribed generically.

PACT level 2 gives more detailed information about practice prescribing costs and the prescribing profile in relation to the six therapeutic groups. As in level 1 a comparison is made between the practice and the average in the family practitioner committee area, but level 2 demonstrates graphically the position of the practice in relation to other practices for various prescribing functions.

55

Prescribing costs

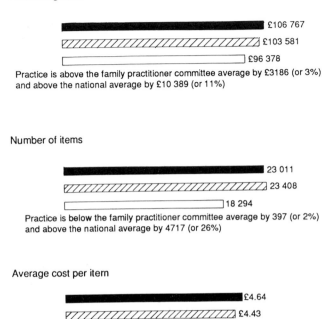

£106 767

£103 581

£96 378

Practice is above the family practitioner committee average by £3186 (or 3%)
and above the national average by £10 389 (or 11%)

Number of items

23 011

23 408

18 294

Practice is below the family practitioner committee average by 397 (or 2%)
and above the national average by 4717 (or 26%)

Average cost per item

£4.64

£4.43

£5.27

Practice is above the family practitioner committee average by 4.7%
and below the national average by (12.0%)

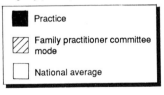

Practice

Family practitioner committee
mode

National average

FIGURE 1—Practice prescribing (PACT Level 1) for quarter ended March 1989.
(*Source*: Prescribing information report issued by Prescription Pricing Authority.)

Further detailed information about the prescribing patterns in
the six therapeutic groups is also provided at this second level
(figure 2).

PACT level 3 produces a much more sophisticated analysis of
the prescribing habits of doctors. All therapeutic groups are
covered using the classification based on that in the *British
National Formulary*. Individual drugs are itemised: the quantities
prescribed, the number of prescriptions, and the cost are all

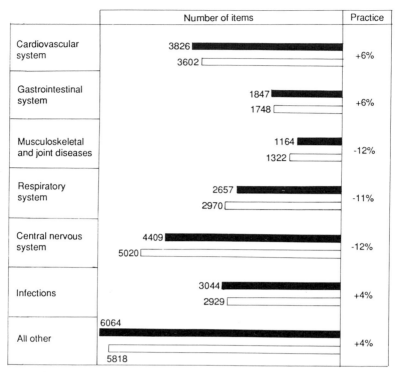

FIGURE 2—Practice prescription items and total cost by major therapeutic group (PACT Level 2) for quarter ended March 1989. (*Source*: Prescribing information report issued by the Prescription Pricing Authority.)

presented in graphic or tabular form (figures 3–5 and tables 1–4).

It can be seen that, with the information available, practices can not only discuss overall practice prescribing trends but also consider variations between partners. This latter exercise can only be carried out successfully if doctors in a partnership always use their own prescription pads, because the information provided by the Prescription Pricing Authority is based on the data from all prescription forms that bear the doctor's identification number. In training practices a trainee practitioner's prescribing figures can be separated out. The trainee needs to write on the trainer's prescription forms only, and endorse the number with the letter D.

A study of prescribing patterns in this depth can produce certain changes in the delivery of primary care. Comparisons will enable partners to look at their prescribing in terms of patient benefit and

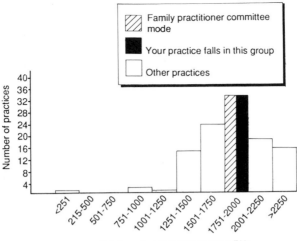

FIGURE 3—Practice prescribing (PACT Level 3) for quarter ended March 1989: distribution of practices in family practitioner committee area by number of items per 1000 PUs. (PUs (prescribing units) based on patients <65 + (patients ⩾65) × 3. As on average patients over 65 receive three times as many prescriptions as younger patients, this factor is included in the expression.) (*Source*: Prescribing information report issued by the Prescription Pricing Authority.)

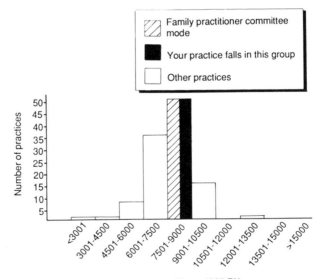

FIGURE 4—Practice prescribing (PACT Level 3) for quarter ended March 1989: distribution of practices in family practitioner committee area by total cost per 1000 PUs. (PUs (prescribing units) based on patients <65 + (patients ⩾65) × 3. As on average patients over 65 receive three times as many prescriptions as younger patients, this factor is included in the expression.) (*Source*: Prescribing information report issued by the Prescription Pricing Authority.)

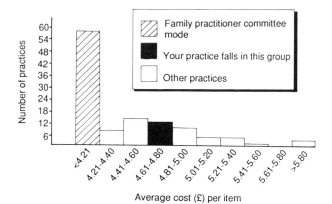

FIGURE 5—Practice prescribing (PACT Level 3) for quarter ended March 1989: distribution of practices in family practitioner committee area by average cost per item. (*Source*: Prescribing information report issued by the Prescription Pricing Authority.)

TABLE 1—Prescribing (PACT Level 3) for quarter ended March 1989: profile

	Prescribing list size	Patients ≥65	Number of PUs	Number of items	Total cost (£)
Doctor	2 806	710	4 226	4 455	22 626
Practice	10 561	1 573	13 707	23 011	106 767
Family practitioner committee average	10 561	1 573	13 707	23 408	103 581

PUs (prescribing units) based on patients <65 + (patients ≥65)×3.
Source: Prescribing information report issued by the Prescription Pricing Authority.

TABLE 2—Prescribing (PACT Level 3) for quarter ended March 1989: analysis by prescribing unit and patient

	Average cost per item (£)	Items per PU	Average cost per PU (£)	Items per patient	Average cost per patient (£)
Doctor	5·08	—	—	—	—
Practice	4·64	1·7	7·79	2·2	10·11
Family practitioner committee average	4·43	1·7	7·56	2·2	9·81

PUs (prescribing units) based on patients <65 + (patients ≥65)×3.
Source: Prescribing information report issued by the Prescription Pricing Authority.

TABLE 3—Prescribing (PACT Level 3) for quarter ended March 1989: percentage of items prescribed generically

	Percentage
Doctor	44
Practice	43
Family practitioner committee	39
National	39

Source: Prescribing information report issued by the Prescription Pricing Authority.

TABLE 4—Prescribing (PACT Level 3) for quarter ended March 1989: extract giving number of prescriptions and cost of drugs in two categories

	Quantity	Number of prescriptions	Cost (£)
Antispasmodic and other drugs that alter gut motility			
Hyoscine butylbromide:			
Buscopan® tablets 10 mg	15	1	0·64
	30	1	1·28
	50	1	2·13
Total		3	4·05
Mebeverine hydrochloride:			
Colofac® tablets (135 mg)	28	1	2·34
	60	1	5·01
	84	2	14·02
Total		4	21·37
Ulcer healing drugs			
Cimetidine:			
Cimetidine tablets 200 mg	56	5	41·55
	84	2	24·92
	450	1	66·75
Cimetidine syrup 200 mg/5 ml	200	1	7·68
Tagamet® tablets 200 mg	40	1	5·93
	56	2	16·62
	120	1	17·80
	200	1	29·67
Tagamet® tablets 400 mg (calendar	56	2	33·22
pack)	60	1	17·80
Tagamet® syrup 200 mg/5 ml	600	1	23·04
Total		18	284·98
Famotidine:			
Pepcid Pm® tablets 40 mg (calendar pack)	30	1	28·50
Total		1	28·50

TABLE 4 (*continued*)

	Quantity	Number of prescriptions	Cost (£)
Ranitidine:			
Ranitidine tablets 150 mg	28	1	13·89
	30	3	44·64
	56	4	111·12
	60	3	89·28
	112	1	55·55
Ranitidine disper tablets 150 mg	80	1	41·67
Ranitidine tablets 300 mg	28	1	25·60
	30	5	137·15
Zantac® tablets 150 mg	28	1	13·89
	30	4	59·52
	40	1	19·84
	56	11	305·58
	60	16	476·16
	90	1	44·64
Total		53	1438·53

Source: Prescribing information report issued by the Prescription Pricing Authority.

cost effectiveness. A detailed study of the figures may lead to the partners making a decision to produce a practice formulary or even, after discussion with hospital colleagues, to consider the introduction of a local combined formulary. It may also show up instances of how hospitals, to protect the drug budgets, may require the general practitioner to prescribe expensive drugs. This will have increasing significance for the doctor with the introduction of indicative drug amounts into primary health care. Audit of prescribing statistics will need to take place at regular intervals so that changes in prescribing habits can be identified.

Hospital referrals

The role of the general practitioner as the gatekeeper to patients gaining access to other services is accepted as an essential part of our health care system, providing a means of identifying patients in need of specialist attention and the method of directing them to the appropriate specialist. Little is known about the factors that prompt a doctor to make a referral and various studies have shown marked variation in referral rates between family doctors.

Wilkin and Smith[4] studied the referral patterns of 201 doctors. They found a marked variation among this small group. They showed that the age, sex, social class, or diagnostic case mix of the patients had little influence on whether a doctor had a high or low referral rate.

Audit of hospital referral patterns within a practice is an important exercise, not only from the point of view of the costs generated but also because these statistics are a terms of service requirement of the practice annual reports to be submitted to the family practitioner committee. The regulations require doctors to submit to the family practitioner committee or health board reports covering the total number of patients referred as inpatients and the total number of patients referred as outpatients. The outpatient referrals are to be categorised according to the clinical speciality and hospital to which the patient has been referred.

Practitioners should arrange for the secretarial staff in their practice to keep a record of all their hospital referrals. The simplest way of doing this is for the practice secretary to record basic details of all outpatient referrals from the hospital referral letters; inpatient referrals, however, will have to be recorded by the doctors themselves. A simple proforma can be devised that will allow the collection of data detailing the number of referrals to the laboratory and x ray departments.

The collation of this information will allow the practice to compile its annual report and will facilitate discussion about differences in referral patterns between the partners. It must be stressed, however, that comparisons of referral patterns within a partnership are meaningless unless consultation rates are also known; even then no definite conclusions about what is good practice and what is bad practice can be made because of the variability of patients' complaints, the characteristics and interests of the doctors, and the availability of open access facilities in the area.

Advantages can, however, be gained from a study of this particular subject. It will enable the practice to take a closer look at the quality of the referrals and the standard of letters that refer the patients to hospital. Indeed, it can be extended to consider the quality of letters received from the hospital and the delay in their receipt by the practice. It may also lead a practice to compare the number of hospital investigations requested with the result of those investigations. It is clear that detailed consideration of hospital referrals may uncover deficiencies in the provision of care and may entice practices to enter into a combined audit procedure with the hospital service.

Out of hours visits

An awareness study of "out of hours" home visits can provide useful information for the practice. It may expose deficiencies in practice organisation; for example, delays in patients being able to see their doctors in normal working hours may cause demands for service in the evening or at weekends. The introduction of the two tier night visit fees under the new contract, combined with an extension of the hours during which they may be claimed (10 pm to 8 am), can also make this a subject of financial importance to the practice.

The data to be collected will be decided by the doctors themselves but probably will consist of the name, address, and age of the patient; the time at which the home visit was requested and when it was made; the reason for the request; and the findings, diagnosis, and action of the doctor who made it. This information will be available from receptionists, caretakers, doctors, patients' families, and deputising and answering services. From this information it will be possible for a practice to identify the workload and the nature of that work in any part of the "out of hours" period, and it will enable the financial implications of any deputising arrangements to be clearly understood.

An audit of an activity of this kind can only be justified if there is benefit to patient care, as well as any possible financial gain. Detailed study may show that patients seek services at these times because they are unable to obtain them during normal surgery hours. This may be due to a previously unnoticed pressure on an appointments system that prevents patients being seen by a doctor within a reasonable time. This organisational problem can be addressed by the practice. The study may, however, reveal that certain patients are seeking to avoid a consultation with their own doctor, or even show up those who are abusing the 24 hour availability of general medical services. The practice will want to rectify this by appropriate patient education and by discussing the problems on an individual basis.

It is probable that partners in a practice might wish to audit "out of hours" visits on a continuous basis or at regular intervals. In noting trends in demand the practice may identify a need for change in its provision. This could involve changes in the use of a deputising service, the extension of an existing rota arrangement, or even the taking on of an extra partner.

Care of the elderly

The terms of service under the 1990 contract expect a general practitioner to offer patients aged 75 years or over a home visit to assess various functions such as mobility, mental state, and continence. Practices will need to have information about this screening procedure, to make certain that it has been done and that any recommendations have been recorded. The age/sex register, whether manual or computerised, will provide the means of identifying the target population; and the simplest possible system can record those patients that have been visited, the findings at the visit, and any deficiencies in provision that have been identified.

Carrying out this audit will ensure that the terms of service are complied with and a dossier of problems of elderly patients compiled. It is anticipated that problems will include housing defects and deficiency in provision of services, such as home helps, household aids, and chiropody. As the yearly assessment of elderly patients is a constant obligation, the practice will have information from successive years and be able to make comparisons about the level of services from year to year. The information so produced will enable doctors to seek better provision for their elderly patients.

The main purpose of this chapter is to consider subjects that could act as a starting point for audit activity. Family practitioner committees have received guidance from the Department of Health in a circular.[5] Practitioners who have taken the basic steps to audit the procedures already described will be able both to understand and to cooperate with the new audit arrangements.

Family practitioner committees have been instructed to establish medical audit advisory groups to direct, coordinate, and monitor medical audit activities within all practices in their area. They have also been asked to ensure that these groups forge appropriate links with those responsible for medical audit in the hospital and community health services so that plans to improve services bridging hospital, community health, and primary care can be formulated.

The members of a medical audit advisory group are appointed by family practitioner committees and include doctors with recognised expertise in, and experience of, medical audit. The majority of the members are practising general practitioners but there is consultant representation to facilitate the bridging exercise. The responsibilities of the groups are fourfold:

(*a*) to institute regular systematic medical audits in which every practice in a family practitioner committee's area takes part;

(*b*) to make certain that adequate procedures are in place to ensure that the results of medical audit in respect of individual patients and doctors remain confidential;

(*c*) To ensure that problems revealed through medical audit are dealt with by remedial action;

(*d*) to provide local management with a regular report on the general results of the audit programme.

It is therefore clear that a practice that has begun its audit of simple contractual obligations will be in a position to contribute immediately to the audit activity in the family practitioner committee's area. As the exercise is being professionally led and conducted on the principle of peer review, practitioners will be able to expand their activities to bring improved services to their patients, creating among the partners an increased feeling of professional satisfaction.

In this chapter the procedures for starting audit activity have been described in some detail. The intention has been to suggest subjects that might be suitable for study in the first instance and how these might be tackled. It has also attempted to show the benefits to patients and practice. These can be summarised as follows:

- Increased personal job satisfaction
- Increased practice efficiency
- Improvement in care of patients
- Compliance with terms of service
- Maximising of income
- Providing a starting point for expanding the audit process into other areas of practice activity, especially those involving the clinical care of patients.

1 Secretaries of State for Health, Wales, Northern Ireland, and Scotland. *Working for patients*. London: HMSO, 1989. (Cm 55.)

2 Department of Health and Social Security. *Medical audit. Working paper 6*. London: HMSO, 1989.

3 Department of Health and Social Security. *Promoting better health: the government's programme for improving primary health care.* London: HMSO, 1989.
4 Wilkin D, Smith AG. Variation in general practitioners' referral rates to consultants. *J R Coll Gen Pract* 1987;**37**:350–3.
5 Department of Health and Social Security. *Medical audit in the family practitioner services.* London: HMSO, 1989.

Chronic conditions

COLIN WAINE

Introduction

Certain chronic conditions are particularly suited to the practice of audit because of their prevalence and because of the nature of chronic disease, which is lingering, stubborn, and more likely to be eased than fully cured. Some chronic diseases and conditions are present early in life—for example, many kinds of handicap. Others appear later in life. A child crippled from birth may never dance; another, congenitally deaf, may never hear music to dance to; someone may become a successful dancer but then fall victim to rheumatoid arthritis and dance no more. Whenever they appear chronic diseases restrict their sufferers' choices and actions; this should be a matter of great concern to their doctors.

Here I deal with five chronic conditions: diabetes mellitus, asthma, angina, chronic handicap, rheumatoid and similar forms of arthritis. The first two sections in this chapter deal with diabetes and asthma in considerable detail to provide the reader with a comprehensive approach to auditing chronic conditions. These provide a full model for the less detailed treatment of angina, chronic handicap, and rheumatoid arthritis. I then consider the audit of palliative care. Since sufferers from any of these conditions may have their ability to work or enjoy themselves impaired, the constant question is: "What can we do to help such patients live as fully as possible in these circumstances?" This leads to the question underlying the last section in the chapter: "What can we do to ensure a peaceful, dignified, and painfree death?" As well as considering audit as a means of monitoring the care we give to our patients with chronic conditions we should also bear in mind what we can do for the quality both of their life and of their dying.

Diabetes mellitus

Diabetes, one of the most prevalent chronic diseases, is a challenge to today's family doctor. There are some 600 000 known people with diabetes in the United Kingdom. In an average practice list of 2250 patients there are likely to be 22 cases of diabetes known to the doctor and another 22 as yet undiagnosed.[1]

Diabetes can occur at any stage of life but its prevalence rises with age. As the average age of the population rises the long-term complications of diabetes are becoming more common.[2] A particular concern for general practitioners is that compared to the rest of the population people with diabetes have twice the risk of a stroke or myocardial infarction, five times the risk of developing gangrene, 17 times the risk of renal failure, and 25 times the risk of blindness.

Despite these known risks for patients with diabetes there is evidence[3] that many general practitioners are not looking after their diabetic patients as well as they should. *Balance*, the patients' newspaper published by the British Diabetic Association, often cites cases of patients knowing more about their condition than their family doctors do.

The requirements imposed on patients in guiding them towards good control are justifiable only if it can be shown that exercising such control will let them live longer with fewer complications. Therefore the following information is important.

A prospective study of 4000 patients between 1947 and 1978[4] showed that complications were worse in those with poor control: there was a higher incidence of complications such as retinopathy, neuropathy, and nephropathy. Good control has a clear inverse relationship with retinal disease.[5] Close control of diabetes can arrest the progress of early retinopathy: patients allowed a freer regime undoubtedly deteriorated.[6] There was no significant retinopathy in people whose blood glucose levels were kept below 11 mmol/l.[7] Retinopathy is also unusual in patients whose glycosylated haemoglobin levels are kept below 10%. The severity and frequency of acute neuropathic attacks are decreased by better control.[8] Triglyceride concentrations in diabetics are directly related to those of glycosylated haemoglobin.[9] This in turn depends on overall blood glucose concentrations over the preceding 6 to 10 weeks. Cataract, a significant complication of diabetes, is undoubtedly associated with poor blood glucose control.[7]

What are our therapeutic aims and standards?

These are our aims.
- To search for diabetes
- To stay in touch with known diabetics
- To control blood sugar within an agreed range
- To search for early signs of end organ damage
- To ensure appropriate actions.

Here we might consider the words of A B Kurtz: "The goals of therapy are set by doctors but have to be achieved by patients."[10]

Our standards follow from the aims set out above.

Searching for diabetes and diagnosing it early and accurately— Diagnosis is not difficult when the patient presents with the classic symptoms of thirst, polyuria, and weight loss. Other signs may be tiredness, pruritus vulvae, balanitis, blurred vision, ulcerated legs and feet (features of neuropathy), intermittent claudication, and recurrent sepsis. If a patient presents with any of these conditions a urine test or blood sugar estimation is indicated.

A fasting blood glucose level of over 8 mmol/l is almost always indicative of diabetes, as is a random blood glucose level exceeding 11 mmol/l. Diabetes is unlikely if the fasting level is below 6 mmol/l and the random level below 8 mmol/l.

Where blood glucose levels lie between these figures a glucose tolerance test can be useful. There is no need to perform the test routinely on patients with symptoms of diabetes whose blood glucose measurements are above 8 mmol/l fasting or 11 mmol/l on a random sample.

The following conditions should be observed in carrying out a glucose tolerance test:
- The patient should have had high carbohydrate meals for three days before the test. If he or she has been ill or has taken prolonged bed rest during this time the test should be postponed
- The test should be done in the morning after an overnight fast
- The patient should not smoke on the day of the test
- The blood glucose concentration is measured fasting, then the patient is given a drink of 75 g of anhydrous glucose in 250 to 350 ml of water and the concentration is measured every half hour for two hours. Some doctors think it enough to measure only the fasting level and the level two hours after giving the glucose. Others prefer three estimations, fasting and one and two hours after the glucose.

Table I shows blood glucose values based on World Health Organisation criteria. More generous values can be allowed in the elderly, especially in women. In this age group the presence of symptoms is more significant than that of seemingly abnormal biochemistry. There is no point in upsetting the life of an elderly person who is asymptomatic and free of complications purely on the result of a glucose tolerance test. Younger patients should be given dietary advice, especially if they are overweight, and should be reviewed periodically. *Pregnant patients must be managed as though diabetic and referred to a clinic specialising in diabetic care.*

Once patients have been diagnosed as diabetic their names must be entered on a register that is regularly updated. If a register is not kept patients will usually be remembered within about six months by the doctor or receptionist, or from a request for a repeat prescription or the patient making an appointment; but that is hardly the way to run an efficient practice.

Staying in touch with known diabetic patients—The diabetes register makes it possible to recall patients regularly. The frequency of recall depends on how well the patient is managing the disorder him or herself; the degree of control achieved; and the presence of other conditions such as infection, neuropathic ulcers, or hypertension, which would demand more frequent attendance.

Controlling blood sugar levels—It is vital to remember that many patients who are not dependent on insulin can be managed by diet alone. For all patients with diabetes, however, diet is an essential part of the treatment.

TABLE I—Blood glucose values based on World Health Organisation criteria

	Glucose concentration (mmol/l)		
Glucose tolerance test	Whole venous blood	Capillary whole blood	Venous plasma
For diabetes mellitus			
Fasting	7	7	8
2 h after 75 g glucose load	10	11	11
For impaired glucose tolerance			
Fasting	7	7	8
2 h after 75 g glucose load	7–10	8–11	8–11

Source: World Health Organisation Expert Committee on Diabetes Mellitus. 2nd report. *WHO Tech Rep Ser* 1980; **646.**

Changing dietary habits is always difficult, and the best way to do it is to start from what the person usually eats. Competent dietiticians can give invaluable help. It is to be hoped that in future they will work much more closely with primary care teams.

In planning a diet the following principles apply to all patients with diabetes.

- The diet should be individually tailored and regularly updated to allow for age, weight, work and hobbies, and ethnic preferences. For non-insulin dependent diabetics and diabetics of normal weight on tablets the diet should provide enough energy for the patient to carry on his or her job and recreations while maintaining an ideal body weight
- In overweight patients the aim should be to reduce the total calories and so achieve ideal body weight (easy to say but difficult to achieve since some people use energy more efficiently than others)
- Increasing consideration is being given to the total energy content of the diet of the patient with diabetes rather than its carbohydrate component alone. (One gram of carbohydrate gives 17 kJ/4 kcal, 1 g of protein the same, 1 g of fat 38 kJ/9 kcal, and 1 g of alcohol 29 kJ/7 kcal)
- Although in the past carbohydrate was quite severely restricted, it is now suggested that it should contribute 50–60% of the energy produced by a patient's diet
- Most of the carbohydrate should be starches rather than sugars, because starches are absorbed more slowly.
- The diet should be high in fibre
- Use of polyunsaturated fats rather than saturated (animal) fats may reduce cardiovascular risk and should be encouraged
- In the light of the information above, a relatively low energy diet can best be achieved by decreasing its fat, sugar, and alcohol content and increasing the proportion of high fibre carbohydrate so that it contributes over 50% of the total dietary energy—for example, by including dried peas, beans, and sweetcorn. Such foods also slow the absorption of carbohydrate after a meal
- Common sense should be applied to the occasional binge, especially with children, for whom there should be ways of judiciously incorporating treats into the diet—for example, a "mini" Mars bar before exercise, or a sweet after a high fibre meal. We are all human.

First we shall consider measures for patients who are not

dependent on insulin. If the patient is *overweight*—that is, 20% or more above ideal body weight—try diet alone for *three months*. Then review the diet and compliance. If control has not been achieved and the fasting blood glucose is above 8 mmol/l add metformin, starting with 500 mg twice a day. (Always check blood urea and serum creatinine first and bear in mind that metformin should not be used in patients with renal impairment, nor for heavy drinkers.) Check control by measuring fasting blood glucose at monthly intervals, always reviewing the diet. If control has not been achieved increase the dose of metformin progressively up to a maximum of 850 mg three times a day. If a month on this dose does not achieve control you should seek specialist help.

Patients should regularly test their urine for glucose and record the results.

If the patient is of *normal weight* try diet alone and review after *one month*. If control has not been achieved, even though the patient complies with the diet, try adding a sulphonylurea drug. *If during the month's trial weight loss continues and/or ketonuria develops earlier review is imperative.* Then review monthly: consider diet and compliance and if these seem satisfactory increase the sulphonylurea in steps to the maximum dose for that particular drug.

Patients should carry out regular urine tests for glucose and if this is above 2%, also for ketones.

If after a further three months on maximum dose control has not been achieved add metformin. If after another three months there is still no control consider insulin injections.

At all the decision points outlined above it is wise to reassess diet and compliance and consider the possibility of infection before changing treatment.

Now we shall consider patients who depend on insulin. The drug can be used in several ways. The three commonest are:
- Two injections of a short and medium or long acting preparation together, morning and evening
- In the elderly, a single injection of a long acting insulin
- A single evening dose of a long acting preparation supplemented the next day by several injections of a short acting one.

In deciding whether it is necessary to adjust the dose of insulin blood glucose monitoring is not only more useful than urine testing in patients suffering from insulin dependent diabetes mellitus but is often more acceptable. For patients on two doses of short and medium or long acting insulin together, if glucose registers too high at one of the following times the basic rules are:

- *Breakfast*—Raise the medium or long acting dose (but also beware of nocturnal hypoglycaemia)
- *Lunch*—Raise the morning short acting dose
- *Evening meal*—raise the morning medium or long acting dose
- *Bedtime snack*—raise the evening short acting dose.

For patients on a single long acting injection, unmixed, base the decision to adjust insulin mainly on the morning blood or urine glucose level.

With the recent trend towards stricter control of blood glucose levels minor hypoglycaemia is inevitably more common. Doctors and nurses looking after diabetic patients should be sensitive to the fears of relatives that the patient may suffer a severe hypoglycaemic reaction. When a patient has an attack of hypoglycaemia the cause should always be sought and discussed with the patient.

The management of ketoacidosis is often a hospital task, but it is within the remit of the general practitioner to identify its cause and discuss this with the patient. The condition is almost always preventable.

Searching for early signs of end organ damage—Check the integrity of the skin. Look for ulceration or infection. Where necessary refer for chiropody. Check the peripheral pulses, dorsalis pedis, and posterior tibial. Examine the eyes for cataract and then, through a dilated pupil, for retinopathy. Once a year check for microalbuminuria or frank albuminuria and monitor the serum creatinine. Check the integrity of the tendon reflexes in the lower limbs and for vibration sense at the ankle. Monitor the blood pressure regularly because the control of hypertension is particularly important in a diabetic patient. Control of blood pressure is second only to control of blood glucose in diabetics.

Ensuring appropriate action—Treat early complications vigorously; for example, treat skin infections with antibiotics and raised blood pressure with appropriate drugs. Make appropriate referrals. For example, if retinopathy is discovered refer the patient to an ophthalmologist; if hypertension cannot be effectively controlled refer the patient to a physician with a special interest in diabetes and hypertension.

Which aspects of performance need to be measured?

We need to know how many patients have had an annual review. We also need to know the proportion of diabetic patients who have had

- glycolsylated haemoglobin measured at least twice yearly
- cholesterol measured yearly or more often if necessary
- creatinine measured yearly
- periodic checks on injection techniques and blood glucose testing, as appropriate.

For each patient we should know

- how often he or she has consulted us
- the number of episodes of hypoglycaemia that have occurred
- the number of times he or she has been admitted to hospital because of ketoacidosis or other diabetic complications
- how many days he or she has lost from work or school through diabetes or related conditions.

We should record the number of diabetic patients with complications affecting, for example, the eyes, feet, kidneys, or cardiovascular system.

What needs to change?

The first need is to review the present state of care in the practice for patients with diabetes, and to decide whether it can meet the aims set out above.

Does the practice have a protocol for the management of diabetic patients? If not is it willing to develop one or to adopt one produced by another group such as the Royal College of General Practitioners?[11]

In the case of particular shortcomings the following five actions are recommended.

(1) If the number of patients on the diabetic register is considerably smaller than would be expected from the age and sex distribution of the population *check the diabetes register once more, using the repeat prescription system.*

(2) If patients are not having eye checks *review the resources available and consider referring them to an ophthalmic optician.*

(3) If control of "diet alone" patients is inadequate *review diet sheets and consider further help from a dietician.*

(4) If data on blood pressure or chest pain are poor *conduct partnership reviews and training of practice nurses.*

(5) If hypoglycaemic attacks are too frequent *review patient education and revise dosage schedules.*

Are all the practice's diabetic patients known and, if so, are their names entered on a register?

Are there facilities for estimating blood glucose, glycosylated haemoglobin, cholesterol, and creatinine?

Can a system be set up for patients to have an annual review? If not can an alternative strategy be devised?

What resources are available or required?

Time—If we are to care properly for patients with chronic conditions, such as diabetes, we have to find time and that time needs to be protected. Some practices have ensured this by setting up a specific diabetic clinic with defined hours. Time has to be protected for two reasons: firstly, it takes a long time to assess the needs of patients and their families and find how to meet them; secondly, professional workers such as nurses, dieticians, and chiropodists need time to meet and pool their skills for the benefit of the patient.

Space—In such a diabetic clinic workers clearly need a protected space of their own, both to carry out their work and to meet.

Records—Proper records are essential for any form of organised care. There should be a standardised record card on which information can be entered in a way that allows it to be easily compared with the findings of previous visits to the clinic. There is much to be said for a system that allows information to be transmitted between primary and secondary care. The patient held diabetes record card of the Royal College of General Practitioners fulfils all these aims. An example of such a card is shown on pages 76–80.

People—The most important person at a diabetic clinic is the patient, who needs the support of skilled and compassionate carers. Ideally these should include a family doctor with a particular interest in the condition, a practice nurse who has developed skills in the care of diabetic patients, a dietician, and a chiropodist. These should in turn be supported by the practice manager and ancillary staff, who can ensure that the appointment system runs smoothly and can chase up defaulters.

THIS IS THE PERSONAL RECORD CARD OF:

Name .... D.O.B. .... M/F

Address .... Tel. No. ....

....

GP. Diabetic Liaison Sister Consultant

Name .... Name .... Name ....

Address .... Address .... Address ....

....

Tel. No......................... Tel. No......................... Tel. No.........................

SIGNIFICANT EVENTS	DATE	NOTES

© THE ROYAL COLLEGE OF GENERAL PRACTITIONERS

FIGURE 1—Antenatal cooperation record card.

Date of Diagnosis ....

PRESENTATION e.g.	Ketoacidosis
	Routine Urine Test
	Recurrent Sepsis

Criteria for Diagnosis

R.B.S.	mmol/l	(> II plasma glucose)
+ /or F.B.S.	mmol/l	(> 8 plasma glucose)
+ /or O.G.TT		
75G 2 hour glucose	mmol/l	(> II)

FIRST EXAMINATION

Height .... Weight .... Ideal Body Weight ....

| URINE | Glucose | Ketones | Protein |

| B.P. | Lying | | Standing |

EYES   R   L

V.A.
Fundi   O   ⨯   ⨯   O

FEET

PULSES	R	L	REFLEXES	R	L	SENSATION	R	L
P. Tib			Knee					
D. Pedis			Ankle					

INITIAL MANAGEMENT PLAN

DIET   OBJECTIVES

TABLETS

INSULIN

FOLLOW UP

Date	Diet	Insulin	Tabs	Loss Work School	Hypos	Inj-Sites	GHb	Notes

FIRST ANNUAL REVIEW   Date.................................

PROBLEMS: WELL BEING:

Smoking   Alcohol   Diet   Hypos

Insulin   Tablets   Photos

EYES   R   L   Date
  V.A.
  Fundi   O   ✕   ✕   O

PULSES	R	L	REFLEXES	R	L	SENSATION	R	L
P. Tib			Knee			Pin Prick		
D. Pedis.			Ankle			Vibration		

B.P.   Standing   Lying
GHb   Creatinine
Changes   Cholestrol
                                               Objectives

FOLLOW UP

Date	Diet	Insulin	Tabs	Loss Work School	Hypos	Inj-Sites	GHb	Notes

SECOND ANNUAL REVIEW   Date.................................

PROBLEMS: WELL BEING:

Smoking   Alcohol   Diet   Hypos

Insulin   Tablets   Photos

EYES   R   L   Date
  V.A.
  Fundi   O   ✕   ✕   O

PULSES	R	L	REFLEXES	R	L	SENSATION	R	L
P. Tib			Knee			Pin Prick		
D. Pedis.			Ankle			Vibration		

B.P.   Standing   Lying
GHb   Creatinine
Changes   Cholestrol
                                               Objectives

78

FOLLOW UP

Date	Diet	Insulin	Tabs	Loss Work School	Hypos	Inj-Sites	GHb	Notes

THIRD ANNUAL REVIEW   Date.................................

PROBLEMS: WELL BEING:

Smoking   Alcohol   Diet   Hypos

Insulin   Tablets   Photos

EYES
  V.A.   R   L   Date
  Fundi   O   ⚬   ⚬   O

PULSES	R	L	REFLEXES	R	L	SENSATION	R	L
P. Tib			Knee			Pin Prick		
D. Pedis.			Ankle			Vibration		

B.P.   Standing   Lying
GHb   Creatinine
Changes   Cholestrol
                                                  Objectives

FOLLOW UP

Date	Diet	Insulin	Tabs	Loss Work School	Hypos	Inj-Sites	GHb	Notes

FOURTH ANNUAL REVIEW   Date.................................

PROBLEMS: WELL BEING:

Smoking   Alcohol   Diet   Hypos

Insulin   Tablets   Photos

EYES
  V.A.   R   L   Date
  Fundi   O   ⚬   ⚬   O

PULSES	R	L	REFLEXES	R	L	SENSATION	R	L
P. Tib			Knee			Pin Prick		
D. Pedis.			Ankle			Vibration		

B.P.   Standing   Lying
GHb   Creatinine
Changes   Cholestrol
                                                  Objectives

FOLLOW UP

Date	Diet	Insulin	Tabs	Loss Work School	Hypos	Inj-Sites	GHb	Notes

FIFTH ANNUAL REVIEW   Date.................................

PROBLEMS: WELL BEING:

Smoking   Alcohol   Diet   Hypos

Insulin   Tablets   Photos

EYES   R   L   Date
  V.A.
  Fundi   O   ✕   ✕   O

PULSES	R	L	REFLEXES	R	L	SENSATION	R	L
P. Tib			Knee			Pin Prick		
D. Pedis.			Ankle			Vibration		

B.P.   Standing   Lying
GHb   Creatinine
Changes   Cholestrol
                                                  Objectives

BRITISH DIABETIC ASSOCIATION

National Address..

....

Local Address ....

....

Patients Notes..

....

....

....

Not all diabetic clinics in general practice will have the services of a dietician and chiropodist, but it should be possible to refer patients quickly. Health districts developing a policy for patients with diabetes should make sure that these facilities are readily available.

Patient and family education—The principles outlined below should be borne in mind.

- Before starting any educational programme define its aims and objectives
- Checklists are useful, but remember that each patient is unique
- Tailor the programme to the patient and not the patient to the programme
- Do not offer too much too quickly: begin with a basic package
- Teaching sessions should not be prolonged; offer the most important items first
- Make full use of literature and teaching aids that can be taken away by the patient and studied at home
- Information from all members of the primary care team should be consistent
- Continue educating the patient.

Equipment—Professionals running a diabetic clinic need the following:

- A register
- A call and recall system
- Record cards
- Booklets for patients to record results of blood glucose monitoring or urine testing
- A good weighing machine
- Snellen test charts for measuring visual acuity
- A good ophthalmoscope, blood pressure machines, and stethoscope
- A tendon hammer
- A tuning fork
- 2% Tropicamide eye drops to dilate the pupil
- Blood glucose testing strips.

Specialised diabetic clinics—Some patients—those with complications such as hypertension, renal failure, and ischaemic limbs—will need the expertise of a specialist clinic. Specialists should be consulted in a spirit of collaboration and not allowed to take over the patient's case. Many people believe that children and pregnant women with diabetes should be looked after mainly by specialist clinics. My own view is that, if they are, they should not lose touch with their general practitioner clinic.

Optometrists—These have skills which can be applied to eye screening for patients with diabetes. Diabetic patients are entitled to free eye examinations if referred by their general practitioner. Optometrists will always agree to examine diabetic patients at least once a year and a regular arrangement can be made for them to do so.

Clinical pathology—Good relationships should be set up with local departments and with the chemical pathologist, and arrangements agreed for all patients to have their glycosylated haemoglobin regularly measured and the quality of their blood glucose monitoring assessed. The clinical pathologist's advice on the interpretation of results can be invaluable.

What is our performance now?

Has a suitable protocol been identified or developed in the practice?

Once the decision has been made to run a clinic, the first task is to identify patients. An up to date disease register makes this simple. If there is none you will have to rely on memory and repeat prescriptions as already described; and this method may miss those patients whose condition is controlled by diet alone and who rarely test their urine. Has responsibility for maintaining and updating the register been given to a specific person?

Have the diabetic patients in the practice been identified and registered? The register should contain 1–2% of the practice population.

Is there a call and recall system for all the patients?

Are those patients who are not dependent on insulin seen at least twice a year and those who are dependent on insulin every four months?

Are the practice ophthalmoscopes suitable for screening? If necessary has training in ophthalmoscopy been arranged for those principals who will run the clinic? Alternatively, have arrangements been made for eye screening by a specialist clinic or local optometrist?

Are the following checks carried out on patients?

(1) At each visit the patient should be asked about problems that

have arisen since the last visit; then the results of blood and urine tests should be studied and the diet and dosage of tablets or insulin reviewed. The patient should be weighed and his or her feet inspected. Blood should be tested for random blood sugar and, if six to 10 weeks have elapsed since the last visit it should be tested also for glycosylated haemaglobin, especially in patients who depend on insulin. Urine should be checked for albumin. Injection sites should be inspected.

(2) Periodic checks may be made on the patient's technique in drawing up and injecting insulin and in testing urine and blood glucose.

(3) Once a year there should be a check of visual acuity and, after dilating the pupil, an inspection of the optic fundus. Also creatinine should be checked each year; so should blood pressure, taken with the patient both lying and standing.

(4) Regular checks on diet by a dietician are highly desirable.

Adequate documentation is essential, both so that findings can be compared with earlier ones and to make the recall system work properly. The Royal College of General Practitioners card has already been mentioned.

There is much to be said for making the patient's next appointment before he or she leaves the clinic.

Ideally, each primary care team should put one of its members in charge of the organisation and smooth running of the clinic.

Practice based diabetic clinics, which deal with relatively small numbers of patients and can offer continuing and personal care, should be highly acceptable to patients and satisfying for the primary care team.

Asthma

Asthma is one of the most important chronic diseases, affecting about 10% of the population. Before this century reliable observers believed that asthma was never fatal but it is now recognised that asthma mortality can be as high as 3 in 100 000 patients each year in some countries. The highest rate is in New Zealand, followed, in decreasing order, by Australia, the United Kingdom, other European countries, and North America.

Recent mortality figures from several countries have shown

disappointingly high rates in those aged between 5 and 34, a range in which diagnosis is likely to be accurate. In the United Kingdom today about 2000 people die annually from asthma and, significantly, more than one third of these are under 55.

Deaths from asthma are not decreasing; in fact they may be increasing. I allow that we still do not fully understand the condition, but I do not think that this is enough to explain why people die from it. Better understanding will no doubt come, but meanwhile we have to find ways of keeping people from dying.

In 1979 a confidential inquiry conducted by the British Thoracic Society suggested that 86% of deaths from asthma could have been prevented.[12] In 1986 a working party of the Royal College of General Practitioners came to a similar conclusion, with a figure of 80–90%

An overall impression from studies of asthma mortality is that patients die because their disease is not properly controlled, and there is much evidence that asthma is underdiagnosed and misdiagnosed.

We have many potent means of controlling asthma. It would be well to consider the words of V M Drury: "Our deficiencies are in the main due not to ignorance of new knowledge but to failure to apply existing knowledge." Nothing, perhaps, exemplifies this better than asthma care. The safe and effective drugs we have had since 1970 for the treatment and prevention of asthma should have improved care for patients with the disorder. We still, however, have a legacy of underdiagnosis, undertreatment, and lack of patient education and proper follow up.

What are our therapeutic aims and standards?

These are our aims:
- To search for and identify all patients with asthma
- To keep in touch with all patients known to have asthma
- To control the asthmatic state so that life is disrupted as little as possible by absence from work or school. Life should be as full and free as possible
- To ensure that patients understand their condition and the aims of treatment
- To let patients know what to do when their condition is deteriorating.

Our standards follow from these aims.

Finding patients with asthma—In diagnosis the main requirement is for the clinician to be aware and suspicious.

Apart from asthma there are few disorders that cause recurrent wheezing in children. Diagnosis should not be hard if a good clinical history is taken, even if the child is not seen during an acute episode. The possibility of an inhaled foreign body, however, should always be considered in a toddler who presents with a first episode of wheezing. A child who wheezes in association with upper respiratory viral infections has asthma, not recurrent bronchitis. Sometimes in children the wheeze is not normally audible, but if, on auscultation of the chest, widespread wheezes are present asthma is probable, as it is when there is a recurrent dry cough at night.

Exercise can often bring on symptoms in children.

In adults the common presenting complaints are of tightness in the chest, wheeze, and dyspnoea. Diurnal variation is a most important diagnostic feature of asthma, symptoms invariably being worst on waking in the morning and being accompanied with a feeling of tightness in the chest. Nocturnal episodes of wheezing are another important feature, but in some patients it is not nocturnal wheezing but nocturnal coughing that is the only symptom of asthma.

Bronchial hyperactivity—an essential feature of asthma—may be reflected in the patient's symptoms. Wheezing and chest tightness may be reported as a response to cold air or smoke. Some may report wheezing in response to drugs, specifically salicylates and non-steroidal antirheumatic drugs. Exercise can induce asthma in adults, but less commonly than in children.

There is no need for the investigation to be elaborate to make a diagnosis. By far the most important procedure is measuring ventilatory function, the most usual way being measurement of peak flow. Isolated or occasional measurements usually do not truly reflect the patient's condition. Far more valuable is a series of measurements obtained by a patient who has been trained to take his or her own measurements of peak expiratory flow rate.

Once patients with asthma have been identified their names must be entered on a register, which is regularly updated. This will at first consist only of newly diagnosed patients. The names of other patients with asthma need to be found from the memories of doctors, nurses, and receptionists; by monitoring repeat prescriptions; and by checking surgery appointment lists.

Keeping in touch with patients who are known to have asthma—The register allows a planned recall system to be developed. No asthmatic patient should leave a consultation without being clearly told when he or she will next be seen. The frequency with which a patient's condition should be reviewed depends on its severity and how well it is controlled, how often acute episodes recur, and the confidence of the patient in managing the disorder.

Controlling the asthmatic state—Adequate control is shown by a series of peak flow readings at or as near normal as possible; the least possible disruption of life, with no absence from work or school, no disturbed nights, no need to cancel social engagements; and in children, adequate growth rate.

Understanding asthma and coping with deterioration—Patients should know that when their symptoms become worse they should immediately start monitoring their peak expiratory flow rate. If this falls to 75% of the predicted value they should increase the use of their steroid inhaler to four times a day (the usual dosage is twice daily). If peak flow rate falls to 50% of the predicted value they should start a course of oral steroids, 40 mg per day for adults and 20 mg per day for children, and contact their general practitioner.

Which aspects of performance need to be measured?

- The number of patients in the practice who are diagnosed as having asthma and are on the asthma register
- The frequency with which patients are reviewed. Are intervals too long or too short? For example, two hospital admissions between review appointments would indicate that the interval is far too long
- Some assessment of each patient's understanding of his or her disorder—that is, whether the patient can recognise deterioration objectively and knows the appropriate action
- Simple measurements such as the number of nights disturbed by asthma attacks; the number of days lost from work or school; the number of courses of oral steroid therapy over a given period (say one year); the number of hospital admissions; how many patients have developed virtually resistant airway obstruction— that is, their peak flow rate cannot be improved by intensive bronchodilator or steroid therapy.

What needs to change?

Primary care teams should take a much more proactive attitude to the diagnosis and management of asthma than the usual approach, which is essentially one of crisis intervention. Asthma should be seen as a notable example of a common disease that, although potentially serious, can and should be managed by the general practitioner.[13]

A primary care team adopting a proactive approach must either develop a protocol for the management of patients with asthma or adopt one produced by another group—for example, that of the Royal College of General Practitioners.[14]

Asthma is thought to affect about 10% of the population. The size of the practice's asthma register should be checked to see if it is reasonably near that percentage of the total register. If not the practice needs to step up the search for patients with asthma, reviewing the clinical criteria for diagnosis mentioned earlier and checking repeat prescription lists.

If patients do not follow your advice on treatment it is probably because they do not understand its aims. If examination of your own notes shows a lack of data on peak flow rates this probably calls for a partnership review and perhaps for the practice nurse to instruct the patient further.

A patient whose asthma is often exacerbated should have a review of how well he or she understands the disorder and complies with treatment. If you can find no fault with his or her understanding or compliance consider obtaining the opinion of a specialist.

What resources are available or required?

The most important resources are an interested and knowledgeable general practitioner and practice nurse. Many patients with asthma can have their condition monitored during ordinary surgery consultations, but there may be something to be gained by setting up a specific asthma clinic.

Such a clinic can be run by a suitably trained nurse; the Asthma Training Society conducts courses for practice nurses.* Little equipment is needed, the most important being plenty of mini peak flow meters. These can not only be used in the surgery but lent to

* Details available from Mrs Greta Barnes, Asthma Training Society, 22 Schollars Lane, Stratford upon Avon CU37 6HE.

patients so that a series of readings can be obtained and treatment or any deterioration monitored. There should also be examples of inhalers so that these can be demonstrated to patients.

There is much to be said for giving patients simple instruction cards giving information such as:

My predicted peak flow reading is . . . If this drops to 75%—that is, . . .—increase the steroid inhaler to four times daily. If it falls to 50%—that is, . . .—take eight 5 mg Prednisolone tablets a day, and contact the doctor. The practice number to ring for an appointment is . . . The practice number to ring for a home visit is . . .

Patient and family education—The principles outlined in the section on diabetes apply equally here.

What is our performance now?

- Has the practice either developed a suitable protocol or identified one that it can adopt?
- Has the practice compiled a register of its asthmatic patients and do the numbers on the register tally with the likely prevalence of asthma in the practice population? Has someone taken clear responsibility for maintaining and updating the register?
- Does the practice have enough peak flow meters and demonstration equipment?
- Are all the patients on the register covered by a planned call and recall system with a frequency suitable for the severity of each person's condition?
- Is each patient's case reviewed periodically and is his or her understanding of the disorder assessed?
- Are the simple measurements referred to on pages 85–6 recorded?

At this stage the practice should move towards auditing outcome. Deaths from asthma are likely to be rare in any one practice but overall their number is still too high, despite the effective measures that are now available to manage asthma. There should be a detailed review of any deaths; if necessary colleagues in secondary care should be involved.

It is in patients' best interests for their asthma to be managed by their general practitioner because he or she can offer better continuity of care than can an outpatient clinic, where they may be condemned to seeing a succession of junior hospital doctors with little experience or understanding of the long term care of their condition.

Angina

Angina is a notoriously unpredictable condition. In the words of G Jackson, "Angina is not a diagnosis to be made lightly, nor a diagnosis to persevere with if there are reasonable doubts."[15] Medical textbooks describe the classical presentation and outline a differential diagnosis, but in the real world of general practice many people present with chest pain that is difficult to diagnose at all certainly. Diagnosis of angina can have a severe effect on a patient's way of life, so such cases must be investigated with great care.

Yet angina is still largely diagnosed according to how the doctor interprets a symptom presented to him or her by the patient. Many patients' angina can be controlled by drugs but some cannot. There is evidence that surgery can lengthen and improve the life of those with coronary disease.[16]

What are our therapeutic aims and standards?

These are our aims:

- To identify among patients presenting with chest pain those suffering from angina
- To provide medical treatment logically and gradually so as to disrupt work and life as little as possible
- To identify those with unstable angina, who need to be rapidly referred for further assessment and possibly surgery
- To identify those whose symptoms are disabling despite maximum medical treatment and refer them for consideration of surgery
- To identify and treat any aggravating factors such as anaemia, thyrotoxicosis, and aortic stenosis and incompetence
- To monitor all patients regularly and ensure that they know when to report significant worsening of their condition.

Our standards follow from these aims.

Accuracy in diagnosis—Practices should have a clear strategy for diagnosing and managing angina. Chest pain suspected of ischaemic origin should be defined from answers to the following questions.

- In which part of the chest does the pain occur?
- Does the pain radiate to other areas?
- What is it like?
- What precipitates the pain?

● What makes it go away?

The site of the pain is usually retrosternal but pain anywhere in the chest aggravated by exertion and relieved by rest should be viewed with suspicion.

The pain may spread to the throat, even into the jaw. Frequently it radiates to the left arm, sometimes to the right, and quite often from a retrosternal site into both arms.

There is often a feeling of constriction and a sensation of heaviness and tightness.

The cause may be anything that raises the demand on the heart, such as exertion, walking against the wind, taking a large meal, going out from a warm room into the cold, or emotion.

Relief is usually obtained by reducing the load on the heart—for example, by standing still after walking, or simply walking more slowly. Pain abates quite soon, usually within five minutes.

Medical treatment—Doctors should be able to rule out precipitating causes such as anaemia and thyrotoxicosis by testing haemoglobin and thyroid function.

Which aspects of performance need to be measured?

● The number of patients suffering from angina, divided into those who are controlled by one, two, and three drugs and those who, in spite of triple therapy, are significantly disabled, and those with unstable angina
● The proportion of those with unstable angina who have been promptly admitted to the local coronary care unit
● The proportion of those not adequately controlled by triple therapy who have been offered referral for further assessment with a view to coronary bypass
● The number of patients with angina who are regularly reviewed
● Whether the practice is kept informed of any developments in the management of angina and coronary heart disease; for example, the criteria for coronary bypass may change and a more interventionist policy may be adopted, as in the United States.

What needs to change?

Practices should take an aggressive attitude to the management of angina, aiming to give their patients the maximum benefit from medical therapy or surgery. It is no longer allowable for patients to be severely disabled by their condition without an offer of referral for further investigation and possible treatment.

Diagnosis must be precise and you may need to refer patients for investigations such as exercise electrocardiography.

What is our performance now?

It is difficult to say how things are on a national scale, but they do not look good. For instance, in 1988 a survey of patients having coronary bypass grafts in the Northern region showed that most of them came from only a few districts. There are variations in the incidence of coronary heart disease in the region but by and large it shares with the North West region the doubtful distinction of the highest rate in England. It seems that in certain health districts too little attention is given to selecting patients who might benefit from bypass grafting—an operation with a high success rate and low morbidity.

Our long term goal should certainly be to lower the incidence of coronary disease by preventive measures, but for those who already have angina more radical steps are appropriate.

Chronic handicap

Here I shall consider a handicapped person as someone who cannot achieve his or her full physical, mental, or social potential. This criterion is adapted from the American Public Health Association's definition of a handicapped child.

What are our aims?

- To prevent handicap where possible—for example, by genetic counselling, more rational prescribing in pregnancy, wider immunisation, and earlier recognition of potentially handicapping diseases
- To develop a plan for early recognition of such diseases
- Full assessment, probably using a multidisciplinary approach
- Immediate treatment where appropriate, as for deafness
- To support the family of the handicapped person
- To continue support for the person and family
- Periodic reassessment
- To arrange vocational training and employment, if possible.

These aims reflect the need to approach the problem as a whole, to recognise handicapped families rather than handicapped individuals, and to keep up care and advice.

What standards follow and which aspects of performance need to be measured?

All handicapped people in the practice should be identified and their names put on a register that is regularly updated.

Each case should be honestly reviewed to see if the handicap could have been prevented and whether it was detected early enough for effective treatment. The degree of handicap in physical, psychological, and social terms should be assessed, as should its cause, diagnosis, treatment, and prognosis. The psychological assessment should extend to the person's family. The social assessment includes the need for special arrangements and services and whether these have been provided.

The nature of the handicap should be carefully explained to the patient, if appropriate, and to the family. People tend to find these things out in a haphazard way from general practitioners and hospitals. The general practitioner needs as much time as possible to explain the matter properly.

If a referral has been made are there good links between primary and secondary care? Referring a handicapped patient does not absolve the general practitioner of responsibility. Referral might also lead to consultation with several doctors in various disciplines, during which it is vital for the general practitioner to see that care is kept up.

Advice to the handicapped and to their families must be consistent; this calls for good teamwork between primary and secondary care.

What needs to change?

General practitioners and primary care teams need to adopt a positive attitude to handicapped people and their families so that they will turn to them for assessment, crisis intervention, advice, and treatment. Patients and their families should feel that they are being treated as individuals and that all available help will be provided.

It is most important for care to be kept up. Balint[17] coined the phrase "mutual investment company" to convey the idea that continuity of care in general practice is like the accumulation by doctor and patient of shared capital, *the capital being the quality of the relationship.*

What resources are available?

The most valuable resource for any handicapped person is a supportive family which, in turn, enjoys the support of a committed primary care team. Specialist help will at times be required and it is essential for the general practitioner to take care in choosing a specialist who has particular interest and skills in the condition.

In many instances it will be appropriate to involve the local social services department, which can provide adaptations to housing. It can also often arrange occupational therapy more easily than can the health service, in which there is a serious shortage of occupational therapists at present.

Sometimes the disablement resettlement officer will need to be called in to secure a suitable job for a handicapped person. It is wise to check with a knowledgeable social worker that the person and family are receiving all the benefits they are eligible for. For families with very young children the health visitor plays a key role. Any family with a handicapped child is entitled to the services of a social worker and on reaching the age of 16 a handicapped person becomes entitled to a social worker of his or her own. Social workers can help the handicapped and their families obtain appropriate benefit payments. They can also help place children in residential homes, where necessary, and arrange relief for families during a crisis or at holiday time.

In certain types of handicap physiotherapy at the earliest possible stage can be vital to the development of good posture, toilet training, and many skills in movement. If there is a problem with speech the local speech therapy department should be called in.

Many areas have community nursing teams dealing with handicapped people of any age. Some children may need home educational services or educational psychologists. Voluntary workers from local associations can also be called in.

What is our performance now?

Over the past two or three decades much more help has been offered to handicapped people but some are still not getting all the information and help they need to make decisions about their future and take advantage of what is on offer.

Voluntary organisations have also grown steadily, which is admirable in itself but a reminder that the needs of certain handicapped people are still not being properly met. Professionals do not always cooperate with voluntary workers as smoothly as they should.

Rheumatoid arthritis

What are our concerns about rheumatoid arthritis?

Rheumatoid arthritis is a widespread condition. Sufferers are often badly disabled and have a great need for skilled help. The disease is neither preventable nor curable; yet, as John Gedney has pointed out, almost all its features can be ameliorated, thus generally improving the patient's wellbeing and morale.

Many disciplines other than general practice can, in their own way, help the sufferer. It is up to the general practitioner to coordinate these, for which task he or she needs excellent knowledge both of the disease itself and of the roles of what may be termed "the rheumatoid arthritis support team."

The disease is variable both in its severity and in its rate of progress. There is no generally agreed set of treatments and even less information on its management in general practice. It does not help that there are still no tests for the disease that could provide numerical data. So the following suggestions for managing rheumatoid arthritis are largely based on the experience of individual general practitioners.

The prevalence of established rheumatoid arthritis in the United Kingdom is usually reckoned to be about 1%. It is two or three times more common in women than in men.[18] If the mildest forms of the disease are included the figure is 2% or even 3%.[19] A general practitioner with a list of 2500 patients will have about 25 with established rheumatoid arthritis and about a quarter of these will become significantly disabled.[20] Two or three new cases might be expected every year.

Scott and Symmons[21] reviewed a series of studies on mortality and rheumatoid arthritis and found that severe rheumatoid arthritis is associated with increased death rates from all causes. All studies report higher death rates from infection and from renal disease, especially amyloidosis.

What are our therapeutic aims and standards?

The overall aim, as in any chronic disease, is that the patient should lead the freest and fullest possible life. The destructive and disabling effects of the disease should be limited as far as practicable, and pain should be relieved to a tolerable level.

The patient should have the full benefit of all the various supporting agencies. To achieve this the general practitioner must retain a principal role in helping the patient and coordinating other helpers.

Our standards follow from these aims.

A diagnosis of rheumatoid arthritis has serious implications for the patient and should be made as certainly as possible—for example, by using the diagnostic criteria set out by the American Rheumatism Association.

Which aspects of performance should be measured?

The first requirement is to identify patients in the practice suffering from rheumatoid arthritis and enter their names on a regularly updated register. Data on the register should allow the general practitioner to assess rapidly the degree of disability of each patient, the helping agencies involved, and the therapy the patient is receiving. It should be clear whether the patient is moving from one category to another—for example, from slightly to moderately disabled—and practical points should be noted, such as whether he or she is still able to work.

Since the drugs used to treat rheumatoid arthritis can have significant side effects data should be kept on them and regularly reviewed.

What needs to change?

Most doctors will need to upgrade their knowledge of rheumatoid arthritis and rheumatic disorders so that they have the best possible diagnostic skills and the knowledge to plan the management of the disorder. The doctor also needs a knowledge of the helping agencies in the district, how to contact them, and how to coordinate their services.

The doctor must also be in close touch with supporting services. It would be a good idea to have a patient held record card to help transfer information between different groups.

The principles by which a patient with rheumatoid arthritis can be managed need to be clearly set out, as follows.

There has to be a strategy for solving as far as possible the problems presented by the patient. In many instances the most pressing problem will be the relief of symptoms such as pain and immobility. The patient also needs to increase his or her autonomy, with the backup of the arthritis support team, and to know about the services available to patient and family.

As in any chronic disease, review should be regular and it should also treat the patient as a whole. Here the control of symptoms is particularly important. Is disability lessening, static, or increasing? Complications of drug therapy should also be monitored.

Any patient with so serious a disease should always have the chance of a further opinion. But whenever a patient is referred the general practitioner should make it clear that he or she intends to keep overall responsibility for the management of the patient, and should seek cooperation with the specialist. General practitioners' skills and constant availability make them best suited to look after patients and their families in the long term. The general practitioner remains in touch with other primary care team members and local organisations that can benefit the patient and has probably known the patient for some years and understands his or her personality and home circumstances.

What is our performance now?

Reorganisation of the care of rheumatoid arthritis on the suggested lines should provide real benefits. Actively seeking sufferers from rheumatoid arthritis and caring for them in the practice is clearly effective. Certain population studies[22] have shown that many patients do not mention such problems to general practitioners of their own accord. Although there will be some patients who need close contact with specialists, most will be best helped by regular and planned care from their general practitioner and primary care team, using specialist advice where necessary. One study[23] showed that patients probably do slightly better, as well as preferring to be looked after, in a clinic that provides structured care.

Palliative care

What are our concerns about palliative care?

Death is the inevitable companion of life, yet today people tend to push it away and speak of it in hushed tones. Therefore it is fortunate that palliative care is a growing branch of medicine. The hospice movement has shown what can be achieved by a positive approach to the terminally ill.

Yet, in 1985, at a conference of the Royal College of Physicians on advanced cancer, Eric Wilkes stated:

A high proportion of patients have ineffectively controlled pain, cough, dyspnoea, and insomnia. There is no room for complacency as there is still a gap between current practice and the optimum in terminal care, irrespective of where the patient is being cared for, and there is still a gulf between the problems perceived by the family, those perceived by the patient and those perceived by the doctor initiating or coordinating care.[24]

Patients with a terminal illness and their families have particular emotional, spiritual, and physical needs. Unfortunately traditional medical training has not always trained doctors and nurses to meet these.

What are our aims?

A man may, by custom, fortify himself against pain, shame and suchlike accidents, but as for death, we can experience it but once and are all apprentices when we come to it.

Montaigne, *Essais*

A peaceful death with dignity and freedom from pain should be the goal of terminal care. The patient and the family must be helped and supported in such a way that the experience allows the family to grow rather than have its integrity destroyed.

Our standards follow from these aims. We must develop
- a relationship between doctor and patient that is based on trust and honesty
- effective support for the patient's carer
- maximum relief of pain and discomfort
- resource, where appropriate, to other caring services such as Macmillan nurses, Marie Curie nurses, and hospice facilities
- respect at all times for the patient's wishes.

Which aspects of performance need to be measured?

It is hard to measure the effectiveness of palliative care. There are no clear criteria.

The mental state of the patient and of relatives is perhaps the best measure of performance; for example, a spiritually upset patient or family is often a sign of mistrust between doctor and patient.

The level to which symptomatic relief is achieved is obviously highly important to the patient. Use of pain charts can be a help here.

The deaths column of the local newspaper can give a clue— "Grateful thanks to the family doctor."

The quality of the relationship between the doctor and the bereaved relatives is most revealing. If he or she is in a partnership do they seek him out for further consultations? A letter of thanks from relatives can be worth a thousand audits. One such letter said, "We are blessed with the best doctors anyone could wish for."

What needs to change?

The first need is for the caring professionals to work out their own attitude towards death. Only then can they develop a style of caring that truly supports patients and their other carers. The approach of "I am sorry, there is nothing more we can do" must not go on. Switching from therapeutic to palliative care should be done positively and not with an air of defeat. Medical science does not have all the answers.

Yet the time honoured systematic diagnostic approach must not be abandoned. Detailed history and careful clinical examination remain most important.

The stages of dying must be understood. Kübler-Ross[25] listed these as denial and depression, anger, bargaining, depression, acceptance. But it should not be assumed that they inevitably come in that order.

It must be acknowledged that some patients will become terminally ill through diagnostic delay or error. If so the anger and antagonism of the patient and family will have to be faced.

Time, commitment, and continuity of care are indispensable. If a peaceful and dignified death is to be achieved relationships have to be effective. Looking after dying patients and their families can be very stressful and this should be acknowledged.

Other disciplines can make a great contribution. Effective terminal care is almost impossible without our community nursing colleagues but others—for example, social workers and occupational therapists—can often play a large role. If the patient is a believer everyone should work closely with the patient's religious adviser.

An updating course on symptom control would be well worth while, as would a study of the useful texts on palliative care, of which there is a growing number. It should then be possible to describe patients' fears of death and dying, to define the stages of death, and to acknowledge one's own attitude to death and the physical, psychological, and social effect of terminal illness on patients and families.

The general practitioner should understand how to communicate with dying patients and their relatives. This will help him or her to make the best use of helping agencies such as the pain clinic, Macmillan nurses, or the hospice. There should also be some understanding of how to prepare relatives for bereavement.

What is the next step?

In palliative care death is not the end. The relatives remain and they need help. Unfortunately our society has no proper way to treat the bereaved and all too often they are shunned.

Perhaps more than anything relatives need to talk, and the primary care team is ideally placed to listen. Relatives should be able to express their feelings openly. They will want to speak of their relationship with the person who has died; if they can now accept his or her bad points as well as the good ones so much the better.

Drugs should be used sparingly, if at all. Often listening is the best medicine.

The primary care team will be able to support most bereaved relatives but they should be on the lookout for abnormal grief reactions and in such cases should not hesitate to call in specialist counsellors. The bereaved need support that prevents life from stagnating at the point of their relative's death, that enables them to go on as individuals, and that helps them to return to a functioning life, though different from that before the loss.

1 Tasker PRW. Is diabetes a disease for general practice? *Practical Diabetes* 1984; 1(1):21–4.
2 Sönksen PH, Judd SL, Lowy C. Home monitoring of blood-glucose. Method for improving diabetic control. *Lancet* 1978;i:729–32.
3 Wilks JM. Diabetes—a disease for general practice. *J R Col Gen Pract* 1973;**23**:46–54; Day LJ, Humphreys H, Alban-Davies H. Problems of comprehensive shared diabetic control. *Br Med J* 1987;**294**:1590–2.
4 Pirart J. Why don't we teach and treat diabetic patients better? *Diabetes Care* 1978;**1**:139–40.

5 Joplin GF *et al. Proceedings of the 7th Conference of the International Diabetic Federation. International Conference 231.* Amsterdam: Elsevier, 1970. (Excerpta Medica International Congress Series No 276.)

6 Kohner EM *et al. Treatment of diabetic retinopathy.* Washington: US Public Health Service publication 1890, 1969.

7 Jarrett RJ, Keene H. Hyperglycaemia and diabetes mellitus. *Lancet* 1976; ii:1009–12.

8 Ward JD, Barnes CG, Fisher DJ, *el al.* Improvement in nerve conduction following nerve treatment in newly diagnosed diabetics. *Lancet* 1971;i:428–30.

9 Peterson CM *et al.* Correlation of serum triglyceride levels and haemoglobin A1C concentrations in diabetes mellitus. *Diabetes* 1977;**26**:507–9.

10 Quoted in Waine C. *Why not care for your diabetic patients?* London: Royal College of General Practitioners, 1988:2.

11 Waine C *et al. Diabetes: a protocol.* London: Royal College of General Practitioners, 1985.

12 British Thoracic Association. Death from asthma in two regions of England. *Br Med J* 1982;**285**:1251–5.

13 Anonymous. Asthma—a challenge for general practice [Editorial]. *J R Coll Gen Pract* 1981;**31**:331.

14 Waine C *et al. Protocol for the care of patients suffering from asthma.* London: Royal College of General Practitioners, 1986.

15 Jackson G. Modern treatment of heart failure. *Modern Medicine* 1989;**2**(20): 32–3.

16 European Coronary Surgery Group. Long term results of prospective randomised study of coronary artery bypass surgery in stable angina pectoris. *Lancet* 1981;ii:1173–80.

17 Balint M. *The doctor, his patient and the illness.* London: Tavistock, 1957.

18 Lawrence JS. The prevalence of rheumatoid arthritis. *Annals of the Rheumatic Diseases* 1961;**20**:11.

19 O'Sullivan JB, Cathcart ES. The prevalence of rheumatoid arthritis. Follow-up evaluation of the effect of criteria on rates in Sudbury, Massachusetts. *Annals of Internal Medicine* 1972;**76**:573–7.

20 Wood PHN, Badley EM. *"If you've got arthritis expert help is badly needed": a report on a survey of the availability of specialists (rheumatologists).* London: Arthritis and Rheumatism Council, 1983.

21 Scott DL, Symmons DPM. *The mortality of rheumatoid arthritis.* London: Arthritis and Rheumatism Council, 1986.

22 Mowat AG, Nichols PJ, Hollings EM, *et al.* A comparison of follow-up regimes in rheumatoid arthritis. *Annals of the Rheumatic Diseases* 1980;**39**:12–7.

23 Lawrence JS. *Rheumatism in populations.* London: Heinemann, 1977.

24 Wilkes E. Terminal care: how can we do better? *J R Coll Physicians Lond* 1986; **20**: 216–8.

25 Kübler-Ross E. *On death and dying.* London: Tavistock Publications, 1970.

Acute conditions

KAY RICHMOND

Acute presentations make up a large part of the workload in primary health care during surgery consultations, home visits, and out of hours calls. The nature, place, and frequency of presentation of such conditions will, in large part, determine the method of audit used. Other variables to be considered are the age and sex of the patients presenting, their disposal—that is, advice, prescription, or referral—and the likely course of the disease. The effects on the practice workload and the usual methods of coping will also need to be examined.

The conditions I shall discuss have been selected to enable examination of different aspects of primary health care and of the interface with the hospital and community health sector. Time scales and contents of the audits will vary with such factors as those mentioned above.

Upper respiratory tract infection

The incidence of such episodes in 1981–82 was 195 for every 1000 people at risk, with an episode rate of 206.9 per 1000.[1] These figures gave rise to a consultation rate of 239.9 per 1000 people at risk with over 20% being home visits. This represents a considerable workload for the practice. Are all these contacts between doctor and patient necessary or desirable for a self limiting illness? If not why not? Can, or should, we attempt to change this pattern? Could the time and other resources used be better spent elsewhere?

Therapeutic and organisational considerations

The incidence of rheumatic fever and acute glomerular nephritis

Dr Kay Richmond is a senior medical officer in the Welsh office. She has written this chapter in a private capacity and the viewes expressed are her own.

were falling before the advent of antibiotics.[2] In 1981–82 the incidence of acute and chronic heart disease, Sydenham's chorea, and acute and chronic glomerular nephritis was 0.3 per 1000 people at risk.[1] It is unlikely that antibiotics have contributed much to this decline. We know that about 40% of upper respiratory tract infections are caused by bacteria[3]; the remainder result from viruses. In 1981–82 follicular tonsillitis and quinsy made up 22.8% and streptococcal sore throat and scarlatina 0.9% of the incidence of such infections.[1] Thus the course of the disease and its outcome are unlikely to be affected by the use of antibiotics in 60–70% of cases. There is evidence that antibiotics do not influence the reattendance rate[4] and that social and psychological factors significantly affect their use.[5] Thus we cannot hope to influence the course or outcome of a large proportion of these illnesses by an excessive use of antibiotics. In addition we teach patients that minor illnesses need a consultation and thus diminish their confidence to manage such conditions themselves, helping to make them dependent on the doctor and unnecessarily increasing the workload of the practice.

Is there any way in which we can adjust these imbalances? An agreed policy on the use of antibiotics—for example, in patients who are toxic or have quinsy—should aim to reduce their use where possible while advice to patients on how to manage upper respiratory tract infections themselves—for example, through the use of paracetamol or aspirin for three days before deciding whether a consultation is necessary—will increase their self confidence and help them to learn how to use the health care services most effectively. This should lead to fewer consultations, enabling the team to free time for other work—child health surveillance, for instance. Such a strategy applied to upper respiratory tract infections and other minor illnesses has been shown to work. In my own single handed practice over the period 1982 to 1987 consultations fell from 5.3 to 4.6 per patient per year, despite vaccination and immunisation uptake levels in excess of 90%, a cervical screening level of 86% (including hysterectomies) in women aged 35–64, and a blood pressure screening level of 95% in adults aged 20–64.[6]

The audit

To determine the current levels of performance in the practice it will be necessary to agree an audit protocol. What will need to be measured and recorded? Who will be responsible for keeping the records? Who will do the analysis and present the results?

Because of the frequency and pattern of occurrence of upper respiratory tract infections it will probably be enough to carry out an audit over only one or two winter months. Since 80% of consultations take place in the surgery it may be easier from an organisational point of view to audit only patients seen there. It may be, however, that the most ill patients are seen at home. Thus to exclude home visits may remove from the audit those most likely to receive and/or need antibiotics. It would therefore be preferable to include all patients presenting with respiratory tract infections over the agreed period.

If the partners agree to put to one side the notes of all patients seen with such infections the collection of data can be undertaken by the practice manager or nurse or one of the partners. An agreed proforma would considerably ease this task.

The data that need to be collected include the following.

- Where was the patient seen and when (surgery, home visit, out of hours)?
- The presence or absence of exudate
- The presence or absence of lymphadenopathy
- The presence or absence of pyrexia
- Was the patient toxic?
- Was a prescription issued?
- If so was it for an antibiotic, antipyretic, or antihistamine, and which one?
- Was self help advice given; if so what?
- How many times was the patient seen for this episode?
- Total practice consulting rate—in surgery, at home, out of hours.

When such data are analysed one can assess the feasibility of reducing prescriptions and increasing self help advice, thus influencing the demand for intervention in future. It may also be possible to consider whether the practice nurse could play a role in managing minor illness.

The lessons learnt

Once the current performance of the primary health care team and patients has been analysed, the use of published evidence should make it possible to consider whether changes are needed. If changes are agreed how can they best be implemented? When the new system has been in operation for a time the audit should be repeated to find out what effect the changes have had. It would be best to carry out this task one year later. Because the second audit would be done at the same time of year as the first, seasonal effects would be removed, although not the effects of an "epidemic" year. The consulting rates for the year ending with the first audit and the subsequent 12 months could be compared to see if there had been any overall effect on the practice workload and if this was beneficial. Prescribing analyses and cost (PACT) data could be used to find the effect on prescribing behaviour. Finally, a value judgment based on the objective evidence will have to be made on the cost/benefit profile of the exercise and the practice's future policy for dealing with upper respiratory tract infection.

Hip, distal radial, and vertebral fractures

This subject heading is intended to show how acute problems can be audited to shed light on the way the team has looked at preventive medicine and the way in which an acute occurrence can act as the signpost to long term problems so that strategies designed to mitigate the effects can be planned.

The incidence of fractures of the neck of the femur, of the distal radius, and of vertebrae has been shown to increase significantly in people over the age of 65, particularly women.[7] Hip fractures are two to three times more common in women than men aged over 35 while Colles fractures are six to eight times more common.[7 8] In 1985, 71% of hip fractures were in women aged over 65, and 3.4% of all hospital admissions for this group were in this category.[7] Of those able to walk before the fracture at least half are unable to do so independently afterwards.[7] Effective rehabilitation could significantly reduce this level of handicap.[9 10] Overall, about 30% of women are at risk of developing an osteoporotic fracture before 90 years of age.[8] Nevertheless, a survey of general practitioners in 1987 revealed that 20% stated that they had never seen a case of osteoporosis.[7] Clearly something is amiss.

Therapeutic and organisational considerations

The screening methods available for osteoporosis are, at present, unsuitable for mass screening programmes. Measurements of bone mass do not differentiate reliably between those who will sustain fractures and those who will not.[7] Thus it is possible to predict the proportion of the population that will develop osteoporosis but not the risk of fracture to the individual. Strategies are therefore needed to reduce the incidence of osteoporosis in the entire population.

The best known method of decreasing the likelihood of osteoporosis in women is the prescription of hormone replacement therapy after the menopause. The effects on the incidence of breast cancer and cardiovascular incidents, however, are not yet fully understood and there is much controversy over the use of the therapy. As many as 50% of postmenopausal women may refuse it since it would mean the return to cyclical blood loss.

Factors other than hormonal ones are known to contribute to osteoporosis. These include body build, immobility, low calcium intake, smoking, and high alcohol intake. Strategies such as calcium supplementation are unproven.[11][12] Many of these factors overlap with other areas of concern in primary health care—for example, hypertension, life style, and dietary habits.

A recent review of osteoporosis published by the Office of Health Economics[7] suggests that the presence of two or more known risk factors in women who have passed the menopause should indicate the use of hormonal replacement therapy. In the review it was estimated that if hormone replacement therapy had been used for the 25% of women most at risk from osteoporosis in 1985 there could have been a 50% reduction in the incidence of hip fractures.

Thus an effective health education and prevention strategy in primary health care may lead to a decrease in the numbers of women sustaining these fractures.

The audit

The loss of bone density is thought to begin after the age of 30,[7] increasing rapidly after the menopause. Fractures are often not presented in the first instance to the general practitioner but are seen initially in the accident departments of hospitals. Therefore to audit this group of diagnoses it will be necessary to institute a system capable of extracting the notes of all female patients aged over 45 who sustain fractures. The practice will usually be notified of these cases by the hospital. If all hospital letters are seen by the doctors in the practice before filing this may simplify the exercise;

otherwise the ancillary staff will need to be fully and carefully briefed.

The incidence of fractures that occur because of osteoporosis is too low for a population approach in all but the largest practices, but a case by case analysis could yield useful lessons in the first instance. Over time, patterns of behaviour will become clearer. In 1981–82 the combined annual incidence of these three fractures was 14.2 per 1000 for women aged 75 or more, 5.9 for women aged 65–74, and 2.8 for women aged 45–64.[1] For a practice of 10 000 patients with 8% of its population being women in the 75+ year age group a total of approximately 11 such fractures could be expected over a period of 12 months. With 10% of the population aged 65–74 six fractures could be expected. With 22% of the population aged 45–64 six fractures could be expected. This gives an expected total of 23 fractures within a year.

The following factors concerning these patients will need to be noted both before and after the fractures occur.

- Age at the menopause (early menopause associated with increased risk of osteoporosis)
- Parity (increased risk if nulliparous)
- Family history (increased risk if mother had history suggestive of postmenopausal osteoporosis)
- Body weight (thin people at greater risk)
- Low calcium and/or fluoride intake (increased risk of osteoporosis)
- High protein intake (increased risk of osteoporosis)
- Smoking, heavy alcohol intake, immobility, steroid therapy (increased risk of osteoporosis)
- Poor vision, mobility, coordination (increased risk of falling).

The presence or absence of any of these factors will need to be carefully assessed to minimise the likelihood of future falls and to halt or decrease the rate of loss of bone mass.

The lessons learnt

The comprehensiveness of the team's health education and promotion strategies, health screening, and the use of the practice nurse and the health visitor may well need careful examination after such an audit. Also the need to involve social service departments will have to be considered. The future care of patients sustaining such fractures will need to be directed towards lessening the effects of the acute episode and the prevention of future falls, fractures, and other disabilities.

Infectious diseases

This audit is intended to show how examining the occurrence of infectious diseases can lead to an assessment of the effectiveness of a vaccination campaign.

During the measles epidemic of 1986 I was puzzled because neighbouring practices were seeing many more cases than I appeared to be seeing. A review of my notifications book for the relevant period revealed five cases, all in children aged 6 to 10 years. Further investigation of these children and of the cohort who should have received measles immunisation over the preceding few years revealed that the cases had all occurred in children who had not been immunised. These included two sisters aged 6 and 7 years whose mother had always failed to bring the children for immunisation and whom I had failed to "catch" opportunistically, and three older children whose immunisation status had never been adequately assessed. The uptake of vaccination in the younger age group was 100%. Thus the pattern of measles notifications was adequately explained and the advantages of a high vaccination uptake were highlighted. A serious failure to assess adequately the immunisation status of children new to the practice was also revealed and corrective steps were taken.

A study of a measles outbreak in an infant school[13] showed attack rates in immunised and unimmunised children of 0.9% and 52.8% respectively. Hastings et al,[14] in a study of a measles epidemic, showed that each child contracting measles was ill for an average of 10.8 days and that the general practitioner spent 26 minutes providing care.

A similar approach could be adopted for flu, except that it is not a notifiable disease and care needs to be taken in any audit that a definition of the diagnosis is agreed and understood by all participants. However, the pattern of a flu epidemic brings it to one's attention rather more quickly than is the case for measles; there is also the advance warning afforded by the World Health Organisation, the Public Health Laboratory Service, the Royal College of General Practitioners' spotter practices, and the spotter schemes in Wales and Oxford. A review of all the influenza cases seen over the winter of 1989–90 could serve to assess the adequacy of application of the programme of vaccination advocated by the Joint Committee on Vaccination and Immunisation in its memorandum.[15] This committee is made up of a panel of experts, representatives of the Royal College of General Practitioners and the General Medical Services Committee and observers from the armed forces and the four United Kingdom health departments.

The audit

Once the cases to be reviewed have been selected from the consultation lists for the period of the epidemic the notes will need to be sifted for the following factors.

- Did the patient belong to one of the groups for whom vaccination is recommended by the Joint Committee on Vaccination and Immunisation?
- Was the vaccine given?
- If so how long before the diagnosis was made?
- If not why not?

The answers to the last two questions may then lead on to organisational matters such as the following.

- Was the vaccination programme completed early enough in the year (for flu) or was the relevant cohort approached systematically (for measles)?
- If not why not?
- If the vaccine was not administered was this because the patient refused it or because he or she was not offered it or because he or she does not belong to a group for whom vaccination is recommended by the Joint Committee on Vaccination and Immunisation?

The lessons learnt

The answers to the above questions may raise such issues as the practice's knowledge of, and application of, the recommendations of the Joint Committee on Vaccination and Immunisation. Although many reasons are traditionally offered for failure to meet vaccination targets, the Peckham report[16] found that the main obstacles to a child's being immunised were the misconceptions among general practitioners about contraindications. This finding has also been reported by Pugh and Hawker,[17] Morgan et al,[18] and Carter and Jones.[19] Surveys of practices to ascertain the prevalence of contraindications have found very few for measles.[20 21] Concerted efforts to increase the uptake have produced rates as high as

97%.[22] Those practices with a team approach had better uptake rates than those where the general practitioner had sole responsibility.[16] In 1989 Liston et al[21] reviewed the performance of their programme and the use of a check list by the practice nurse; only one contraindication (to pertussis) was found in 155 cases and the check list allowed the smooth operation of the clinic run by nurses.

It would appear that where the practice is well organised and the Joint Committee on Vaccination and Immunisation recommendations are known and comprehensively applied the uptake of vaccination and immunisation programmes can reach the recommended WHO targets. This would significantly reduce mortality and morbidity levels for the diseases covered and reduce the workload of infectious diseases for the primary health care team. Another perspective is offered by monitoring infectious diseases, particularly in epidemic years, as a means of assessing the effectiveness of the practice's vaccination and immunisation programmes.

Abdominal pain

Abdominal pain is a frequent presentation in primary health care. In 1981–82 the incidence of this non-specific label was 28.2 per 1000 patients at risk[1] with 9.2% of patients seen being referred to hospital, 2.7% as inpatients. An audit by Edwards et al[23] showed that 89% were managed entirely in the practice, 15% were investigated by the practice, 11% were referred to hospital, while only 2% were true surgical emergencies.

Abdominal pain requires careful history taking, examination, and investigation, with referral to hospital as appropriate. The chain of events presents a number of areas for audit that will lead to examination of the role of the patient, the practice team, and the hospital service. Grace and Armstrong[24] found that agreement on the reason for referral between patients and general practitioners was only 49.3%, between consultants and general practitioners 48.8%, between consultants and patients 47.8%, and between all three parties 33.3%. Clearly there is much room for improvement in communication between all concerned.

Therapeutic and organisational considerations

The causes of abdominal pain are legion, extending from acute appendicitis to cholecystitis, renal colic, urinary tract infection, ectopic pregnancy, strangulated hernia, and many others. As well as diagnostic pitfalls there may be problems of delay in the patient seeking help, problems in contacting the doctor, overbooked and rigidly organised appointment systems, unhelpful reception staff, inadequate history taking and examination, inadequate investigation, and inappropriate treatment or referral. Edwards *et al*[23] found that the median figure for days of pain prior to consultation was two. There may be undue delay in obtaining the results of investigations or in finding a hospital bed, or long outpatient waiting lists and delayed or inadequate hospital replies. Mageean[25] found that just over half the patients discharged from hospital had seen their general practitioner before he or she had received any information and that the content of communications was variable with important subjects often omitted; no communication was received for 11% of discharged patients. All facets of the process require careful examination.

The audit

Because of the frequency of presentation of abdominal pain a prolonged audit period will not be needed. Three months will probably be enough. The notes of all cases occurring within the period will need to be identified by the doctors. If a proforma has been designed and agreed for the audit the practice nurse or manager can then obtain the information required. The following points will need to be included in the proforma.

- Time from the start of the illness to consulting the doctor
- Reason(s) for any delay(s)
- Investigations undertaken and their results
- Time between requesting or doing investigations and receiving the results
- Presumptive diagnosis
- Confirmed diagnosis
- Disposal method—prescription, advice, referral as inpatient or outpatient, request for domiciliary visit
- Reason for referral
- Ease or difficulty of referral
- Result of referral
- Time from referral to receipt of reply
- If admitted time from discharge from hospital to receipt of report
- Outcome of episode.

The lessons learnt

Review of this audit will cover many areas. In cases where the patient has delayed seeking advice the reasons will need to be explored. These could range from "I didn't want to bother you doctor" through difficulties in reaching the surgery, either by transport or telephone, overbooked appointment systems with no room for emergencies, to unhelpful receptionists. Organisational hurdles will have to be examined and ways of removing them explored. The practice leaflet may need to be rewritten so that instructions for contacting the surgery in emergencies are clear and concise. Appointment schedules may need to be changed to free time for possible emergencies—for example, leaving a number of appointments unbooked until the previous surgery or having a combination of appointments and "join the queue" arrangements. Receptionists who are too protective of their doctors may need to have their energies redirected with explicit instructions given on how to deal with urgent requests. Perhaps the attitude of the doctor needs adjustment: it may be that the receptionist is "piggy in the middle" between an irascible employer and a desperate patient.

The investigations undertaken, if any, will depend on the provisional diagnosis. For example, where there was doubt of a urinary cause was a urinalysis undertaken? If not why not? Were labstix and/or a microscope available? What was the result of the investigation? Were appropriate actions taken as a result? If there was time to request hospital investigation what was the time between the request being made and the test being done? How long did it take for the result to reach you? Were the results helpful? Were the tests requested or done appropriate?

The presumptive diagnosis will need to be checked against the definitive one for accuracy. If there was disagreement what was the reason for it? Was the difference within reasonable limits? If not what lessons can be learnt?

If advice and/or prescriptions were given were they appropriate? Did they achieve the desired result? Might there have been a better way of proceeding? Did the treatment have any side effects?

In the case of hospital referrals the ease or difficulty in obtaining help will need to be known. If there was undue delay or difficulty should this be pursued with the relevant authorities?

The outcome of all referrals will need to be known. If the patient was admitted was the care satisfactory? Was a definitive diagnosis made? How long was the patient kept in? How promptly were you notified of discharge? What were the discharge arrangements? Was the discharge appropriate (for example, adequate care being available at home) and was the district nurse involved? If so was the level of care appropriate or adequate? In the case of elderly and disabled people it may have been appropriate to involve the social services department. After an inpatient admission or an outpatient referral a letter summarising the hospital's activities and the opinion of the consultant should be received. How long did this letter take to arrive? Were its contents comprehensive and relevant? Any areas of concern about the hospital's performance will need to be pursued with the consultant or management as appropriate.

At the end of the exercise we should be able to judge the outcome for the patient, the practice team, and the hospital and community health sector. Collation of all the facets discussed should be undertaken at the end of the audit and underlying patterns discerned. There is little point in undertaking such a thorough review unless the shortcomings and deficiencies revealed are rectified and a repeat audit done after an appropriate interval to ensure that the lessons learnt have been applied and all concerned have benefited.

Urinary tract infection

Doctors in primary health care are frequently presented with symptoms of urinary tract infection. Cystitis and unspecified urinary tract infections (but not glomerular nephritis, pyelonephritis, or pyelitis) occur in 22.5 per 1000 patients at risk.[1] Women were involved five times more often than men with the age of peak incidence being 15 to 44 years when the ratio of males to females was approximately 1 : 12. This peak coincides with the period of greatest sexual activity and of childbearing.

Therapeutic and organisational considerations

The most common presenting symptoms are dysuria and frequency, 50% of cases being associated with bacterial urinary tract infection.[26 27] Most of these infections are due to *Escherichia coli*, and trimethoprim is probably the antibiotic of choice.[26] In half of these *E coli* infections spontaneous cure can be expected within 72

112

hours.[26] Before writing a prescription one has to decide which cases are likely to be bacterial in origin.

The patient's discomfort is usually severe enough for there to be considerable pressure for an immediate diagnosis and treatment. Labstix and side room microscopy can be helpful.[26] Alternatively, the diagnostic methods described by O'Dowd et al[28] or Dobbs and Fleming[29] may be used. If a mid-stream urine specimen is taken it should be sent to the laboratory immediately or stored at 4°C until despatch is possible. Once a decision to issue an antibiotic has been taken the length of course will need to be considered and may vary between one and seven days.[26] However, 5–10% of infected patients will remain bacteriuric. Whether or not a prescription is issued appropriate advice on follow up and management of possible future episodes should be given.[27]

The audit

The collection of data will need to be made over a six month period and should cover the following points.
- Duration of symptoms before presentation
- Presence or absence of dysuria, frequency, nocturia, and incontinence
- Presence or absence of proteinuria and haematuria
- If a microscope is available the numbers of cocci and white blood cells in each high power field should be recorded
- Whether a pretreatment urine specimen has been sent to the laboratory
- Result received from laboratory on pretreatment specimen
- Advice given (verbal or written)
- Prescription given (which drug, dosage, duration)
- Follow up arranged
- Follow up attended
- Follow up urine specimen sent to the laboratory
- Result received from laboratory on follow up specimen
- Appropriateness of prescription
- Outcome.

The lessons learnt

Once again delays in presentation need to be considered. Can these delays be ascribed to the patients or to the practice? What can be done to minimise them in future?

The correlation between symptoms, diagnosis, management,

and outcome should be examined. Were appropriate investigations carried out? Were the collection, transport, and examination of specimens satisfactory? If the results of hospital investigations were not received by the time of the patient's follow up visit the reasons for this will need to be explored and negotiations with the appropriate people should be initiated to improve the service.

The Public Health Laboratory Service and other microbiology laboratories keep records of the results of all tests submitted. It would be useful to have regular updates of the results, particularly the organisms grown and their antibiotic sensitivities. If these updates are not already being provided it may be worth investigating the possibilities for the future; for example, it may be possible for a quarterly or annual update of the numbers and proportions of all specimens sent by general practitioners (urine samples may account for 40% of bacteriological specimens and samples submitted by general practitioners 10% of the overall workload)[28] together with a summary of the results to be circulated by the family practitioner committee.

If advice on self help and prevention were not given why not? Appropriate patient literature may be obtained and handed to the patient during the consultation and displayed in the waiting room.

Accurate, timely, and caring management of urinary tract infection needs to be ensured to minimise the risk of recurrence and long term complications.

Acute diarrhoea

The majority of cases of acute diarrhoea seen in British general practice are caused by viruses.[30] In 1972 in England and Wales 297 children aged less than 1 year died of acute diarrhoeal disease— more than any other EEC country except for Italy.[31] By 1984 the numbers of deaths from intestinal infection for this age group had fallen to 30.[32] The incidence of severe dehydration and hypernatraemia have been greatly reduced, probably because of the introduction of low solute milks and oral rehydration therapy. In contrast there has recently been an increase in the notification of food poisoning—13 124 cases in England and Wales in 1985 and 20 363 in 1987.[33]

Therapeutic and organisational considerations

In 1981–82 the combined incidence of intestinal disease of proven and presumed infective origin was 34.2 per 1000 people at risk[1]; this gave rise to a consultation rate of 43.9. Of these patients 0.7% were admitted to hospital, 0.5% were referred to outpatient departments, and 0.1% were referred to accident and emergency departments.

In 1979–80 and 1982–83 Kumar and Little[34] carried out two surveys of children admitted to hospital with gastroenteritis. The use of drugs dropped from 50% to 16% between the two surveys, and of those admitted 83% received oral rehydration in the first survey and 94% in the second. The children treated with drugs before admission needed to stay in hospital for longer. Another hospital survey in 1987–88[35] showed inappropriate treatment with drugs in 17% of cases and that 18% were not following the recommended guidelines for feeding during acute gastroenteritis. During hospital admission 88% were treated with standard oral rehydration solutions. A diagnosis of the post-enteritis syndrome was made in 11% of children but all resolved satisfactorily within four months on a diet free of cow's milk and lactose.

Diarrhoea may be prolonged in a small percentage of patients. It may be due to the following factors:

- Post-enteritis syndrome
- Salmonella or shigella; treatment with antibiotics is rarely needed and should be given only after expert advice
- Campylobacter; treatment with erythromycin may be necessary
- *Giardia lamblia* or cryptosporidiosis; it may be necessary to use metronidazole
- Other causes; for example, typhoid fever if the patient has recently been abroad.

Any case suspected of being contracted from food or water will need to be notified to the medical officer of environmental health so that the source of infection and contacts can be traced and measures taken to limit the spread of the infection. This is of particular importance with the current increase in food borne infections thought to be due to inadequate storage and handling. These infections may also be attributed to food being stored for too long in fridges and freezers, to inadequate hygiene, and to failures in food preparation, such as food being cooked for too short a time.

Most cases of acute diarrhoea are seen and managed successfully in general practice, but you will need to know if the management has been appropriate.

The audit

The audit will need to take place over a period from three to six months. Because of the various ways in which patients may come to the notice of the health care team the notes of all patients with a relevant diagnosis (diarrhoea and vomiting, gastroenteritis, dysentery, etc) seen in surgery and at home by the doctor or nurse will need to be kept to one side for completion of the agreed proforma. In addition the post will need to be sifted in order to spot patients coming to light through hospital letters, from occupational health services, and the medical officer of environmental health.

The data requiring collection should include the following:

- Place of presentation
- By whom seen
- Symptoms and signs
- Laboratory specimens and the results
- Advice given
- Treatment given, if any
- Medical officer of environmental health notified—yes/no
- Removed from work if a food handler—for example, cook, waitress, children's nanny?
- Hospital referral. Why, where, type?
- Outcome.

The lessons learnt

Analysis of the above data should enable you to answer such questions as these.

- Is our consultation rate for this problem high, average, or low? Are there any explanations?
- Was the patient seen by the appropriate person—nurse, doctor or hospital?
- Was there delay in presentation; if so why?
- Were appropriate specimens taken?
- Was appropriate advice given?
- Was appropriate treatment given, if any?
- Was hospital referral appropriate; what was the management there; was a timely and relevant letter received?
- Was the medical officer of environmental health notified? Degree of liaison and outcome
- Were the process and outcome the best that could have been achieved? If not why not?

The particular points to be noted should include the appropriate use of staff, the appropriate use of oral rehydration therapy, the inappropriate use of antidiarrhoeals, antiemetics, or antibiotics, and appropriate or inappropriate referral to hospital and/or notification of the medical officer of environmental health.

A repeat audit during the same months one year later will reveal if proper advice on oral rehydration therapy has, as well as being better for the patients, enabled greater patient autonomy and self confidence in handling minor illness with more appropriate recourse to the primary health care team where the course of the illness has been atypical or protracted, thus helping to utilise the team's resources more effectively and efficiently.

Summary

I have tried to show how the audit of acute conditions can be the route to wide and far reaching examinations of subjects rather than of the index conditions in isolation. The wider areas I have attempted to cover are appropriate prescribing, factors affecting workload, screening, acute conditions leading to chronic ones, health promotion and education, appropriate laboratory tests, appropriate hospital referrals, adequate communication between the primary health care team and the hospital and community sector, vaccination and immunisation performance, and the interface with public health medicine. The types of audit covered should help you to examine the structure, process, and outcome of primary health care in your practice so that you may gain increased health and autonomy for your patients and greater job satisfaction for yourselves.

1 Royal College of General Practitioners, Office of Population Censuses and Surveys, Department of Health and Social Security. *Morbidity statistics from general practice: third national study. 1981–1982.* London: HMSO, 1986.
2 Irvine DA. The general practitioner and upper respiratory tract infection in childhood. *Family Practice* 1986;3(2):126–31.
3 Marcovitch H. Sore throats. *Archives of Diseases in Childhood* 1990;**65**:249–50.
4 Howie JGR, Hutchinson KR. Antibiotics and respiratory illness in general practice: prescribing policy and workload. *Br Med J* 1978;ii:1342.
5 Howie JGR. Clinical judgement and antibiotic use in general practice. *Br Med J* 1976;ii:1061–4
6 Richmond JK. *The feasibility and cost of a screening and treatment programme for hypertension in general practice.* Part II project for the Faculty of Community Medicine. (In libraries of the Faculty of Public Health Medicine and the Royal College of General Practitioners.)

7 Griffin, J. *Osteoporosis and the risk of fracture.* (Current Health Problems No 94.) London: Office of Health Economics, 1990.

8 Cooper C. Osteoporosis—an epidemiological perspective: a review. *J R Soc Med* 1989;**82**:753–7.

9 Kennie DC *et al.* Effectiveness of geriatric rehabilitative care after fracture of the proximal femur in elderly women: a randomised controlled trial. *Br Med J* 1988;**297**:1083–6.

10 Currie CT. Hip fracture in the elderly: beyond the metalwork. *Br Med J* 1989;**298**:473–4.

11 Kanis JK, Passmore R. Calcium supplementation of the diet—1. *Br Med J* 1989;**298**:137–40.

12 Kanis JK, Passmore R. Calcium supplementation of the diet—II. *Br Med J* 1989;**298**:205–8.

13 Kimmance KJ. A measles outbreak associated with an infants' school. *Health Trends* 1989;**21**:40–1.

14 Hastings A *et al.* Measles: Who pays the cost? *Br Med J* 1987;**294**:1527–8.

15 Joint Committee on Vaccination and Immunisation. *Immunisation against infectious disease.* London: HMSO, 1990.

16 Peckham C, Bedford H, Senturia Y, *et all. The Peckham report. National immunisation study: factors influencing immunisation uptake in childhood.* Horsham: Action Research for the Crippled Child, 1989.

17 Pugh EJ, Hawker R. Measles immunisation: professional knowledge and intention to vaccinate. *Community Medicine* 1986;**8**(4):340–7.

18 Morgan M *et al.* Parents' attitudes to measles immunisation. *J R Coll Gen Pract* 1987;**37**:25–7.

19 Carter H, Jones IG. Measles immunisation: results of a local programme to increase vaccine uptake. *Br Med J* 1985;**290**:1717–9.

20 Kemple T. Study of children not immunised for measles. *Br Med J* 1985;**290**:1395–6.

21 Liston A *et al.* Use of a contraindications checklist by practice nurses performing immunisation at a well child clinic. *J R Coll Gen Pract* 1989;**39**:59–61.

22 Anderson PMD. Measles immunisation: what can we achieve? *Update* 1987;**1**(9):408–12.

23 Edwards MW *et al.* Audit of abdominal pain in general practice. *J R Coll Gen Pract* 1985;**35**:235–8.

24 Grace JF, Armstrong D. Reasons for referral to hospital: extent of agreement between the perceptions of patients, general practitioners and consultants. *Family Practice* 1986;**3**(3):141–7.

25 Mageean RJ. Study of "discharge communications" from hospital. *Br Med J* 1986;**293**:1283–4.

26 Brumfitt W, Hamilton-Miller JMT. The appropriate use of diagnostic services: investigation of urinary infection in general practice: are we wasting facilities? *Health Trends* 1986;**18**:57–9.

27 Pill R, O'Dowd TC. Management of cystitis: the patient's viewpoint. *Family Practice* 1988;**5**(1):24–8.

28 O'Dowd TC *et al.* Sideroom prediction of urinary tract infection in general practice. *The Practitioner* 1986;**230**:655–8.

29 Dobbs FF, Fleming DM. A simple scoring system for evaluating symptoms, history, and urine dipstick testing in the diagnosis of urinary tract infection. *J R Coll Gen Pract* 1987;**37**:100–4.

30 Nicholl A, Rudd P (eds). *Manual on infections and immunizations in children.* Oxford; Oxford University Press, 1989.

31 Anonymous. More about infant diarrhoea [Editorial]. *Br Med J* 1977;ii:1562.

32 Office of Population Censuses and Surveys. *Mortality statistics: review of the*

Registrar General on deaths by cause, sex and age in England and Wales, 1987. London: HMSO, 1989.

33 Office of Population Censuses and Surveys. *Registrar General's annual returns, 1987.* London: HMSO, 1980.

34 Kumar GA, Little TM. Has treatment for gastroenteritis changed? *Br Med J* 1985;**290**:1321–2.

35 Jenkins HR, Ansari BM. A hospital survey of gastroenteritis in South Wales. *Arch Dis Child* (in press).

36 Wharton BA *et al*. Dietary management of gastroenteritis in Britain. *Br Med J* 1988;**296**:450–2.

Clinically significant events

GRAHAM BUCKLEY

Introduction

Audit is a mean, pernickety kind of word which is inadequate for the imaginative, stimulating activity which it seeks to describe. European general practitioners have preferred the term "quality assurance," which has a more positive ring to it. This chapter considers clinically significant events and so focuses on the heart of general practice—the consultation.

The only requirement for this type of audit is positive motivation by the doctor. No specialist registers or sophisticated information systems are needed, only the wish to become involved because of the realisation that we can all improve our clinical skills.

The field is a wide one: all consultations between doctors and patients are of clinical significance to at least one of the participants; furthermore, this chapter covers the whole of general practice. Concentrating on single clinical events is a simple and practical method of selecting important aspects of practice for scrutiny. One type of audit examines the processes of care associated with clearly defined outcomes—for example, births, deaths, emergency admissions to hospital, and adverse drug reactions. Another fruitful approach is to select consultations at random.

Medical audit is usually taken to mean an exercise involving the collection of quantitative information about groups of patients or about patterns of intervention within a health care system. This has been the main thrust of medical audit over the past 10 years.[1] The objectivity of this approach is commendable, but the relevance of quantitative information is doubtful if not placed in the proper context; for example, to make any judgment about the number of referrals by general practitioners to gastroenterologists it is necessary to know morbidity patterns within the practice, the availability of open access contrast radiology and endoscopy, and whether general physicians in the locality also see patients with gastrointestinal problems.

Restricting audit to aspects of medicine that are easily quantifiable and measurable excludes large and important areas of clinical practice. The medical anecdote has rightly fallen into disrepute as a valid way of advancing an argument about the best way in which to manage clinical conditions. The special circumstances and idiosyncrasies that are present in an individual case may preclude any general inferences being drawn. Nevertheless, the audit of single cases and single consultations is important in identifying issues that can be pursued and tested in other settings and on other occasions. More than other types of medical audit the analysis of single cases and single events defines and refines questions rather than providing answers.

I start my examples of medical audit of clinically significant events with random case analysis because it is a simple technique that reaches the core of general practice. General practice is unique in medicine in having no fixed boundaries. Our clinical work is determined by what patients think is appropriate to present, reveal, or hide. Random case analysis samples the whole breadth of general practice and permits audit to be vigorous yet open ended and open minded. I began this introduction by bemoaning the connotations of the word "audit." We must take care to prevent the reality of medical audit from becoming censorious, negative, and dispiriting. Provided that it is carried out with honesty and sensitivity in cooperation with trusted colleagues the audit of clinically significant events will be sustaining and invigorating and consequently likely to be integrated into general practice to the lasting benefit of both doctors and patients.

Random case analysis

This approach to the evaluation of clinical skills has become established as a major element in the training of general practitioners. At its simplest the method requires just a list of patients seen at a recent surgery session. At a tutorial between a trainee and trainer it is the custom for the trainer to select a case from the list at random and question the trainee about it. The trainer and the trainee may learn more from this activity if from time to time the procedure is reversed and the trainer is questioned about his or her management of cases.

In a group of trainees, in a Balint group, or other small discussion groups the technique can be adapted so that each participant brings a list of patients or agrees to describe the patient seen at a previously specified time—for example, the third patient seen on a Tuesday morning.

This simple technique is a robust and powerful method of revealing the way in which doctors consult but it depends on how the individual doctors perceive the consultation.[2] This inevitably biases subsequent discussion and evaluation. Audio and video recordings of consultations are free from this kind of bias but do introduce possible intervention effects into the consultation itself. The mechanics, acceptability, and evaluation of video recording consultations have been extensively described and discussed because of the unrivalled possibilities the technique provides for evaluating and learning interviewing skills. Although well established as part of vocational training, random case analysis is not yet a normal part of continuing medical education for general practitioners. Balint groups pioneered the use of routine clinical material as the basis for learning about the way in which patients and doctors interact. These groups continue to prosper but involve only a small number of self selected general practitioners

Many general practitioners still seem reluctant to expose their consultation behaviour to the scrutiny of those with whom they work. Part of the reluctance may relate to the paradox which lies at the heart of clinical medicine. As scientists doctors learn to be sceptical and critical about current conventional wisdom and to keep open minds about the efficacy of therapeutic interventions; but as clinicians they discover the benefits of giving patients confidence in their diagnostic pronouncements and treatment recommendations. Apparent clinical confidence becomes part of the armamentarium of general practitioners, who nevertheless remain aware that this confidence does not rest on a solid foundation and can easily be punctured by peer review. Introducing random case analysis into continuing medical education needs to be done with care and tact. If this is achieved the rewards in terms of job satisfaction and improved team work could be immense.

An important principle to be adopted in all forms of random case analysis is to look for positive features before negative ones. The doctor under scrutiny should be given the first opportunity to describe the consultation and note the good features before commenting on the weaker aspects. Similarly, the trainer or peer group when discussing the case should also first identify good points rather than areas of weakness. Specific criticisms should be offered only when a better approach can be suggested. This procedure may seem to be excessively protective of the sensibilities of experienced professionals but it is all too easy to concentrate in a destructive way on one small, weak aspect of a consultation that is otherwise effective.

Whatever method of random case analysis is used the types of questions asked will be similar.

Has the clinical problem been clearly identified?—Why has the patient come? Why today? Why to this particular doctor? These related questions are the starting point for understanding the consultation and are implicit in the opening remarks made by the doctor to the patient. The opening comments by doctors and patients are crucial in determining the way in which consultations proceed, and are likely to reflect previous encounters. Byrne and Long[3] showed how doctors can become stereotyped in their opening remarks in consultations. This may not matter if the remarks are welcoming but otherwise neutral and permit patients to raise issues in the way they wish.

It is possible to discuss at length the possible reasons for a patient's consulting a particular doctor on a particular day. The reasons may be purely pragmatic and relate to constraints within the practice organisation. Questioning along the lines outlined above, however, may alert the doctor concerned to aspects of the consultation that had not previously been considered. It may place the content of the consultation in the appropriate context and influence the way in which the doctor starts his or her consultations in future.

Have underlying or continuing problems been declared or explored?—In the currently fashionable jargon the doctor and the patient may each have an agenda for the consultation that is not explicit at the outset and not part of the presenting problem. General practitioners are familiar with consultations in which patients reveal major health problems or worries just before they leave. During consultations patients are assessing doctors and may use a relatively trivial health problem to judge whether the doctor may be willing to respond to other health problems. Video and audio recordings of consultations are the only way in which any judgment can be made about a doctor's ability to pick up clues about underlying health problems. The recording may reveal moments when the doctor could have offered the patient the opportunity to present additional health problems.

Stott and Davis[4] provided a model for the consultation that has received widespread acceptance. In this model, in addition to the management of the presenting problem, consultations can also include the management of chronic problems, opportunistic screening, and health promotion. Not every consultation will include these aspects of the doctor's agenda but if the pattern that emerges from random case analysis is for a doctor to concentrate exclusively on the presenting problem of the patient this area of questioning will challenge him or her.

What are the expectations of the patient from the consultation? —Doctors tend to assume that they know what patients expect from consultations and consequently they fail to check them out— for example, more patients receive antibiotics for sore throats than expect them. An important element in the consultation therefore is to clarify the expectations of the patient. Audio and video recording may show ways in which this aspect of the consultation is successfully dealt with and illustrates the way in which this technique is a powerful educational tool for observers as well as the observed.

There has been recent interest in the concept of health beliefs. Deeply embedded attitudes concerning health appear to influence the way in which people use health services. Patients who rarely if ever see their doctor appear to have a strong sense of their own wellbeing and resilience; other patients may be basically pessimistic about their own health and bring transient symptoms and minor health problems to the doctor for consideration. Random case analysis may reveal whether the doctor can place the present consultation in the context of the health career and health beliefs of the patient.

Do we have adequate information about the clinical problem?—Other questions are subsumed under this question such as: What investigations are required? Has a sensible treatment plan been formulated and explained adequately to the patient? In these aspects of a consultation doctors will feel more secure and confident since they directly relate to the training they receive. Elsewhere in this book emphasis is given to the creation of standards of care and the criteria by which health care is judged. It is true that in many clinical conditions, such as diabetes, epilepsy, or hypertension, standards of care can be established. One of the goals of clinical medicine is to establish standards of care on the basis of evidence and research. Much of general practice remains uncertain. Patients present with symptoms, not with diseases, and, in the absence of certainty, treatment may have to be on the basis of probabilities about the possible causes of symptoms or even just at the level of symptom relief.

For example, conventional standards for the management of urinary tract infection could be: adult women complaining of dysuria and frequency should have a pretreatment specimen of urine tested bacteriologically; treatment should be on the basis of the sensitivity of the identified pathogen; and a sample of urine taken after treatment should be tested to demonstrate eradication of the infection. In practice there are difficulties with these standards. Mid-stream specimens of urine are not infallible in diagnosing urinary tract infections. The delay between the onset of symptoms and the identification of the infecting organism may be intolerable for some women, who may request immediate treatment with antibiotics. The general practitioner may feel that the balance of benefit lies in complying with this request and selects an antibiotic on the basis of local patterns of infection. In a personal audit of my management of suspected urinary tract infection in adult women less than 10% of the patients handed in specimens after treatment. Women who no longer have symptoms of dysuria and frequency do not have a strong incentive to hand in a further urine specimen. Population surveys indicate that up to 5% of women have asymptomatic bacteruria. Population surveys also indicate that most women with symptoms of dysuria and frequency initially seek advice from a pharmacist rather than a doctor and only if symptoms persist for more than two or three days do they seek the advice of a general practitioner.

Perhaps a more sensible set of criteria for the management of women complaining of dysuria and frequency in general practice is as follows.

- Is there anything about the case that alerts the doctor to potentially serious problems? Is this a recurrent problem? Could the patient be pregnant? Is there a family history of renal problems? Does the patient have other health problems that may make the possible urinary tract infection potentially more serious (for example, diabetes)?

● Are there identifiable precipitating factors affecting the condition (for example, relationship to sexual intercourse)?

An audit evaluates whether a search for these features was carried out by the doctor. Other criteria can be advocated. Some doctors consider that it is important to have objective evidence of infection before treatment. They would wish to have the microscope examination of urine as a criterion of good care.

The difficulty in creating criteria of good care extends to many of the common conditions seen in general practice—for example, sore throats, earache, and respiratory tract infections. Although absolute standards of care cannot be set because of deficiencies in our basic knowledge and in our diagnostic abilities, we are still obliged to develop clinical policies that are sensible, consistent, and coherent. It brings no credit to the profession or to a particular practice if the treatment offered for these conditions varies according to the day of the week or with the particular doctor consulted. Audit exposes uncertainty as well as measuring performance against established standards.

How did the doctor feel about the consultation?—It is important in the analysis of a consultation for the doctor under scrutiny to be given the opportunity to describe how he or she felt about the consultation as a whole. Dissecting the consultation into its component parts is useful but the overall impact of the consultation should not be neglected. Consultations which technically may be deficient may nevertheless be worth while because of the empathy, genuineness, warmth, and concern displayed by the doctor. This is not to minimise criticisms of technical aspects of the consultation, but a consultation may be technically competent and yet be deficient in these general qualities. A patient who leaves a consultation believing that the doctor has taken an interest in his or her problem and is genuinely concerned in seeking a solution will be likely to return and provide the doctor with further opportunities of helping. A cool, detached doctor may only have physical problems presented by the patient, who may choose not to reveal important psychosocial dimensions to his or her problem.

Random case analysis is an important technique in medical audit as it demonstrates that all aspects of medical care are available for scrutiny. It is a necessary counterbalance to the view that much of general practice is amenable to the implementation of protocols. Each consultation is rich in human potential. The spark of genuine communication between a patient and a doctor may be ignited over apparently banal medical problems. We must guard against crushing spontaneity, imagination, and creativity in consultations because of external requirements to document, categorise, and report on their content.

In the rest of this chapter I look at different types of clinically significant events. The selection is idiosyncratic and arbitrary and starts with an event that is unlikely to figure in medical textbooks.

Heart lift

There have been several papers that have sought to define "heart sink" patients—patients whose name on a surgery list evokes gloomy anticipation on the part of the doctor. In pursuing the theme that audit should be about positive aspects of general practice as well as negative ones we need to draw attention to consultations that have a positive outcome for the doctor. Descriptions of these patients can be an enjoyable lead into random case analysis.

There is also a serious aspect to this exercise. In general practice doctors are likely to see 30 or more people each day. There is the danger of consultations becoming routine for the doctor so that the problems of patients are dealt with at a superficial level only. Or there is the opposite danger that general practitioners become overwhelmed or "burnt out" by the emotional needs and demands of patients. The antidote to these dangers is the humour, excitement, surprise, and uplift which consultations also produce. These motivating and energising feelings will be reinforced by sharing them with colleagues.

In the next section we consider more conventional clinically significant events by examining life events.

Life events

Births—In a list of 2000 patients there are likely to be over 20 births each year. Fortunately major obstetric problems are now rare and quantitative audit will be unlikely to be rewarding. Recording the number of mothers who breastfeed their infants is worth while as a measure of the effectiveness of health education in the antenatal period. Detailed questioning of some or all of the mothers will provide qualitative information that might identify strengths and weaknesses in the care provided by the practice. Mothers may be more forthcoming to the midwife or health visitor than to the doctor and communication between the different members of the team could establish criteria of care against which information from the patient could be matched; such communication also identifies areas of care that cause concern for members of the team—for example, smoking during pregnancy. One way of formulating the aims of antenatal care are given below.

- The mother understands the purpose of antenatal clinics in identifying risk factors for delivery and in assessing the progress of her pregnancy
- The mother knows what to expect at different stages of labour and what action to take
- The mother is aware of the benefits of breast feeding and of how she can be helped to initiate breast feeding
- The mother knows how to seek help and advice about herself and the baby in the puerperium.

These have been set out as a list of objectives for the mother's knowledge and understanding since these can be ascertained by interviews with the mother in the first month after delivery of the baby.

If the audit has been jointly planned by the different members of the primary care team it is more likely that information gathered will then be acted on by the team. An audit by one profession in isolation could be seen as threatening by the other professions involved.

Marriage—Marriage is not yet seen in this country as a reason for visiting the general practitioner. Although a happy event, marriage is accompanied by changes in lifestyle that may be stressful. Notification of a change of name through marriage is an opportunity for a general practitioner to suggest a consultation to discuss family planning, provide preconceptual advice for the couple, and check whether the young married woman is immune to rubella.

Death—Less than a third of people die in their own homes and not all of the people dying at home suffer from illnesses that involve terminal care. On the other hand, many of the patients who die in hospices or in hospitals will have been cared for by the primary care team during their final illness. Research studies have shown areas of weakness in the services provided by primary care to the terminally ill and their carers. These weaknesses relate to the way in which information is provided and the inadequacy of symptom relief, especially pain control. Sensitively handled analysis of the care provided for the terminally ill can be of benefit both to the surviving relatives and to the primary care team. Feelings of guilt and anger are normal components of grief and these feelings may be present in all who cared for the dying person. Enlisting the help of the bereaved person could be therapeutic for the individual as well as beneficial for the service. Aspects of care that the bereaved carer could be asked about include the following:

- Frequency of visits by the general practitioner, district nurse, specialist nurse
- Continuity of care
- Symptom control—pain, bowel function, mental distress
- Communication with the patient, with relatives, within the health care team, and with specialist colleagues
- Timing of referral to hospital.

Suicide—Death by suicide is by any reckoning a clinically significant event. Suicide leaves a legacy of distress in the family of the dead person and a sense of failure in the health workers involved. Acknowledging and sharing these feelings in a discussion within the primary health care team will help the doctors and nurses cope and equip them to help in turn the relatives of the dead person. An honest evaluation of the factors leading to the suicide is necessary. There may have been extensive support given to the patient extending over many years, or even more tragically the suicide may appear to have been a sudden impulsive action by someone apparently well. Medicine and doctors do not have a monopoly of relevant skills. The spiritual dimension to this event is obvious and the involvement of a minister with the family and with the practice team may be welcomed. Guilt and forgiveness seem a long way from resource management and audit, but general practice is a long way, thank goodness, from the retail trade.

Medical emergencies

Chest pain—Each general practitioner is likely to be called to one or two patients each year who are suffering from acute myocardial infarction. A similar number of people will be seen who are suffering severe acute chest pain but who do not have myocardial infarction. Acute chest pain is a potentially life threatening event and it is important for practitioners to be able to respond quickly and effectively when informed about a patient suffering from severe chest pain. The precise arrangements for responding to such a call will depend on geographical and other factors, but the following check list will help to establish whether the practice can respond appropriately.

- Practice switchboard not overloaded; incoming calls answered quickly
- Telephone receptionist aware of the need to be able to respond quickly to a patient suffering chest pain
- General practitioner available and able to respond immediately to the call; contact procedure understood by reception staff
- Appropriate equipment and drugs immediately accessible.

This form of audit can and should be carried out without having to wait for the next emergency. Most of the delay between the onset of symptoms of myocardial infarction and treatment is due to the patient. Delay in treatment has an adverse impact on the prognosis after myocardial infarction. The development of thrombolytic agents in readily injectable forms emphasises this point. Practices will need to decide whether to stock them, and whether to have portable oxygen sets and carry electrocardiograph and defibrilator machines. The quality of the local ambulance service and the proximity of the coronary care unit will influence the decision of the practice.

In reviewing the management of a case of myocardial infarction the procedures carried out can be reviewed and any weaknesses identified. Another important function in reviewing the case, however, is to determine whether there were any avoidable risk factors for the heart attack. Had the patient's blood pressure been checked? Was his or her smoking status known? Had the weight been checked in the past three years? Was there a strong family history? Following successful initial treatment of a person suffering a myocardial infarction, what assessments were made to help the patient achieve a return to full function? In attempting to minimise the risk of further attacks, is the lipid status of the person known and has the possibility of familial hyperlipidaemia been ruled out?

Epileptic fits and febrile convulsions—General practitioners are likely to be contacted when a patient suffers a first seizure. Although epilepsy as a chronic problem is common in general practice the number of people experiencing first epileptic seizures is only likely to be one or two a year for each general practitioner. A practice may also expect to see one or two febrile convulsions.

The response of the practice to patients who present with their first seizure is considered in this chapter. The management of epilepsy as a chronic problem would follow the guidelines set out in the chapter on chronic conditions, though it is is not specifically mentioned there.

There are a number of areas of possible concern surrounding the management of a first seizure. These include: management of the seizure itself; accuracy of the diagnosis and identification of possible causes; the understanding of the patient and his or her carers about the seizure and its implications for work and leisure activities; and the compliance of patients with recommended treatment regimes.

Analysing the way in which an emergency call is received may reveal different problems at different times of the day. Having received the call the doctor needs to be able to respond quickly and have available the appropriate drugs. Reviewing the clinical management of a seizure is likely to lead to a discussion between the partners in a practice about the best drugs for use in this situation. Agreeing a clinical policy, even if this policy specifies a range of drugs from which the individual doctor can choose, is a useful step if it leads to ensuring that these drugs are immediately available to the duty doctor.

After successful management of the seizure a decision has to be made whether to refer a patient to hospital. A number of factors will influence this decision; for example, in the case of a child a prolonged seizure and the absence of focal signs of infection would favour immediate referral to hospital because of the possibility of meningitis. An adult suffering a first seizure on withdrawing from heavy alcohol intake might not require immediate referral.

Justifying the particular decision made in a particular case helps to make these criteria explicit and so develops a practice clinical policy. It is this aspect of case review that makes the audit of clinically significant events an educational process for the doctors involved. Other aspects of the early management of seizures that can be included in a practice policy include the types of investigations to be carried out and whether to offer prophylactic therapy to patients after a first seizure.

Another important element in management is to check the understanding of the patient and relatives of the problem and its implications. The possibility of repeated seizures means that driving, unsupervised swimming, and other potentially dangerous activities must stop. Coming to terms with these changes in lifestyle may be difficult for some people and medical audit includes an evaluation of the way in which patients and their relatives react. Conventionally, the review of individual cases tends to rely on the written case record and the memory of the doctor concerned. There may be opportunities for inviting the patient to join in the review of the case. Alternatively, the views of the patient or the parents of a child who has had a febrile convulsion may be presented by means of a video recorded interview.

New diagnosis of malignant disease

The diagnosis of malignant disease is undoubtedly a major clinical event. The commonest neoplasms in men are lung cancer and large bowel cancer. In women carcinoma of the cervix and breast cancer are the malignancies we are most likely to see. Taking all cancers together a general practitioner is likely to see about three new cases each year.

The areas of potential concern surrounding the diagnosis of malignant disease include avoidable factors, delay in diagnosis, communication with patient and relatives and with other agencies involved in care, and responsibility for continuing care. Many of the avoidable factors and delay in diagnosis may lie in the domain of the patient, with cigarette smoking and denial of symptoms common factors in men and avoidance of cervical cytology screening in women. Nevertheless, the occurrence of cancer, particularly carcinoma of the cervix, will cause a practice to question whether its health promotion and screening programmes are sufficiently active.

Questions in each of the categories listed in the box will be helpful in evaluating all clinically significant events.

- Avoidable factors
- Delay in response
- Intervention
- Communication
- Rehabilitation

In the case of malignant disease it is worth questioning whether the treatment offered to a patient was discussed adequately, in particular whether different treatment options were discussed with him or her. How the information about the diagnosis of malignancies is conveyed to the patient and to relatives merits inquiry. Surveys suggest that many patients are not given a clear description of the nature of the cancer and are left to speculate on the extent of their problem.

HIV disease

The diagnosis of HIV infection poses problems for patients that are similar to those of malignant disease, with the added problems of stigma and the effects on sexual relationships. The first case of HIV infection in a practice provides the opportunity for educating the whole of the practice team. This can be achieved while maintaining confidentiality at the level requested by the patient. Many patients infected with HIV have shown themselves willing to discuss with health professionals the way in which they became aware of their illness and the effect that it has on them.

HIV tests need to be carried out in a variety of circumstances. Applicants for life insurance and for visas for some countries are sometimes required to have the test done. Increasingly people who think that they may be at risk of infection because of high risk sexual activity, intravenous drug use, or accidental exposure through injuries are asking for the test. In all cases people need to be aware of the implications of a positive and of a negative test. A review of a particular case would seek to establish whether enough information had been given to the patient before the test was done. Whatever the result of the test the patient needs to understand the need to avoid high risk behaviour in the future. In behavioural terms therefore a test is irrelevant and an individual may prefer the uncertainty of not knowing their HIV status to the certainty of a positive test. The provisional results of treating infected people at an early stage in their disease with zidovudine, however, indicate that there may be a practical benefit in confirming the diagnosis of HIV infection.

Before carrying out a test for HIV a policy on the way in which information about tests is to be handled within the practice should be established. Doctors, medical secretaries, and nurses should all be aware of the way in which test results are received and recorded. After discussion the practice may agree not to share information about a patient's HIV status.

All staff should be aware of the ways in which HIV can be transmitted, in particular the fact that the virus cannot be spread through normal social contact. A practice meeting about HIV infection is an opportunity to tighten up on clinical activities involving invasive procedure and on the way in which equipment is sterilised.

Counselling after the test has been done cannot be completed in a single interview. Patients who are found to have the antibody for HIV will be stunned when they are first told, and their capacity to take in additional information will therefore be limited. A second consultation is essential, and efforts should be made to ensure that the patient has the support of friends or relatives as he or she adjusts to the information. The prognosis needs to be given in a realistic manner, but this does not mean being unduly pessimistic. Many people remain well for many years and there have been significant therapeutic advances. Monitoring the level of CD4 lymphocytes, along with other features, provides a good prognostic assessment. The value of continuing supervision should therefore be emphasised. Before the test, counselling about social behaviour should be reinforced for the HIV positive person. Whether other people should be informed requires careful consideration. Sexual partners do need to be told, but unless the occupation of the patient involves putting other people at risk—for example, if the patient is a surgeon—there is no overriding need to inform anyone else. The extent to which information about a patient's HIV status should be shared within the practice team needs to be discussed explicitly. In an emergency it may be to the advantage of the patient if the duty doctor is aware of the HIV status, otherwise the diagnosis of *Pneumocystis carinii* pneumonia may be missed or delayed.

The House of Commons Social Services Select Committee stated that the care of people with HIV infection is important in itself but will also act as a guide to the adequacy of our health care system as a whole. General practice should be a major contributor in the care of people with HIV infection and AIDS. To make this contribution we need to demonstrate our willingness to participate, to develop clinical expertise, and to learn how to link with the specialist services and voluntary agencies that are already providing much of the care for these patients.

Sudden onset disability

A stroke or a fall resulting in a fractured femur is an event which transforms the life of one of our patients. Strokes and fractured femurs are common clinically significant events, but because in most cases the early weeks of treatment are in hospital the crucial importance of primary health care for these patients is not sufficiently recognised. Surveys have revealed the sorry plight in which many disabled elderly people often find themselves after they are discharged from hospital. An audit of the rehabilitation of these patients will necessarily cover the whole range of community services. The particular contribution of home helps, physiotherapists, health visitors, occupational therapists, district nurses, and general practitioners will vary from individual to individual. Much effort often goes into the multidisciplinary assessment of these patients before they are discharged, but it is rare for a systematic review of them to take place one to two months after they have left hospital.

Discharge from hospital could act as the trigger for an audit exercise in which all elderly people in a practice who had been discharged from hospital in the previous six months could be reviewed in a systematic way. The check list below shows the areas that the review might cover. Medical audit tends to focus on the performance of doctors and other health workers; it can also evaluate the availability of resources. The audit may reveal that the major deficiency in the care of disabled older people is in the lack of resources in the community. Medical audit then becomes a means for lobbying the health and social service authorities; for example, the physical needs of disabled people may be being cared for adequately but loneliness is found to be a feature common to all the patients reviewed. This could support the case for providing transport to day centres for the elderly.

The following check list might be used for assessing elderly people.

- Mobility and balance, indoors and outdoors
- Self care and continence—bathing and toileting
- Social support—relatives, neighbours, home help
- Nutrition—meals, teeth
- Mental status—mood, memory
- Foot problems
- Vision
- Hearing
- Medications—compliance, non-prescribed
- Finance—benefits
- Housing—hazards
- Review arrangements—general practitioner, health visitor, district nurse, frequency.

Referrals to a hospital

The new contract for general practitioners requires practices to provide information on the use made of hospital facilities. For budget holding practices the cost as well as the number of hospital referrals will need to be calculated. The government is interested in this aspect of general practice because three quarters of health service expenditure relates to the hospital services. Surveys have repeatedly demonstrated that there is a wide variation in the number and in the pattern of referrals made by general practitioners. The variation is reduced but still considerable if practices rather than individual practitioners are used as the denominator in calculating referral rates. Variations between doctors are not associated with any identifiable factors such as age, qualifications, or experience. Other than as a fiscal exercise simple quantitative analysis of the use of hospital services is unlikely to illuminate the quality of practice. To learn from analysing referrals to hospital it is necessary to place the quantitative data in the appropriate context. The use of hospital based facilities for investigations in general practice is considered in the next section. This is done to show how simple audit projects can be undertaken while at the same time demonstrating how difficult it is to draw any inferences about quality of care from the data.

Investigations

The simplest quality control type of audit projects in general practice assess the way chronic illness is monitored. For the patient this is not a clinically significant event and is considered in the chapter on chronic diseases. Most other investigations are, however, of clinical significance to the patient. The investigation indicates that the patient and/or the doctor considers that it is important to test for a possible physical cause for the problem presented by the patient.

Haematology, biochemistry, simple contrast radiology, endoscopic examinations, and computerised tomography are examples of diagnostic services that may be directly available to a general practitioner. In the United Kingdom these services are usually hospital based.

The request for a full blood count is a common event in general practice and can serve as a model for the audit or more elaborate investigations. The basic questions for an audit project in this area are as follows:

- Can criteria be agreed within the practice concerning the appropriate use of the haematology service in carrying out full blood counts?
- Can data be gathered on all requests for full blood counts from the practice?

After discussion partners may agree on criteria similar to the following:

- It will be possible to state a reason for requesting a full blood count (a) in the anticipation of a normal result and (b) in the anticipation of an abnormal result
- The test result, whether normal or abnormal, will have an impact on the subsequent clinical management of the patient
- Procedures for informing the doctors and patients of the test result will be reliable
- Partners will have similar ratios of abnormal to normal test results.

The practical procedure may be conducted along the following lines. The haematology department may be able to identify the source of samples for full blood counts by the practice and doctor. The laboratory is likely to provide only samples numbers, but new computer facilities may make possible the identification of individual patients. The laboratory may be able to state whether the total number of requests is similar to that from other practices of equivalent size. More precise comparisons of numbers of requests may be possible by agreement with other practices.

It is helpful if the practice keeps a register of all samples sent to hospital laboratories. This is useful for checking the date of despatch of samples and other data that may enable a missing result to be tracked down. From the register it will be possible to calculate the number of requests for full blood counts made by each doctor over a period of two months. This length of time is chosen because it is likely to identify about 30 requests by a particular doctor and within the short time period doctors may be able to recall details of the consultations not recorded in the patient's notes.

For each request for a full blood count the doctor is asked the following questions:

- Was the request made at the first or at a subsequent consultation for the presenting problem?
- Reason for the request?
- Was the test expected to be normal or abnormal?
- Did the result influence subsequent management of the patient?

Experience from previous studies indicates that it is likely there will be considerable variation between doctors in any group practice in the number of requests made. Suppose that in a five doctor practice Doctor A arranged for 60 tests of which 16 were abnormal and Doctor D arranged for 15 tests of which 8 were abnormal. In all the cases both doctors thought that the test results influenced their subsequent management of the patients.

In the absence of other information it would be easy to draw the erroneous conclusion from this data that Doctor A is profligate in his use of laboratory investigations and that Doctor D may be missing some cases of anaemia in the patients he sees. At a simple operational level there may be factors that contribute to the difference in pattern between the two doctors. Doctor A may conduct most of the antenatal clinics in the practice and be required to send blood for full blood count as part of the overall local clinical policy on antenatal care; Doctor D may only consult in the afternoons when access to the haematology laboratory is difficult.

Nevertheless, these figures are likely to be the starting point for a discussion within the practice about the workload of different doctors, the case mix of patients seen by different doctors, and the threshold for investigation for different doctors. In the absence of quantitative data it is difficult for doctors to discuss how they respond to patients with ill defined symptoms such as feeling tired. Audit of this kind does not demonstrate that the doctors with high or low rates of investigation are right or wrong in their clinical practice. All doctors who participate in this type of clinical review are stimulated to question their own patterns of behaviour and are given the opportunity to learn from the ways in which other doctors manage common clinical conditions.

Clinical mistakes

Earlier in this book (pages 1–14) Marshall Marinker highlights the need for doctors to learn from their mistakes. Error in clinical medicine is inevitable. Our knowledge of disease, physiology, and human behaviour will always be less than perfect, as will our knowledge of our own strengths and weaknesses.

Each year a general practitioner is consulted between four and 10 thousand times and the average length of a consultation is less than 10 minutes. The range of problems brought to a general practitioner is wide. Consequently, in spite of high volume, the number of patients with a particular disease is small and it is difficult to maintain technical expertise in a specific area of practice. These characteristics of general practice mean that errors will be frequent and they should be regarded as normal. As yet, however, errors have not been regarded as an important resource for medical audit or continuing education.

Fortunately most errors in general practice are not dramatic or life threatening but this does not diminish their potential value in indicating ways in which clinical practice can be improved. Honest discussion of a perceived clinical mistake could not only prevent a recurrence of the error but also reveal systematic problems within a practice that require tackling.

Before giving examples of the ways in which clinical mistakes can be utilised in medical audit it may be helpful to explore the barriers to this type of audit. No one enjoys admitting to error. This innate reluctance is compounded in medicine by our early clinical training. Public humiliation on teaching ward rounds soon convinces the more sensitive medical student that the most important skill is not to avoid error itself but rather to avoid the exposure of error. This lesson may be reinforced when as a house officer the most pressing requirement is not to help patients but to keep consultants happy by providing them with cosmetic versions of the truth. This is an overstated description, but it is fair to say that there is no active encouragement in medical education to learn from the inevitable errors that occur.

There is a need to separate error from blame. Blame and the fear of litigation are a barrier to our learning from our mistakes. Anything that goes wrong in medicine is now seen as the basis for legal action. This is damaging in the long run for patients and for doctors. Attempting to prove medical negligence is difficult, lengthy, and costly for patients. Fear of litigation may lead doctors to overinvestigate their patients and focus attention unduly on physical aspects of ill health.

For medical audit into clinical mistakes to prosper a climate has to be created in which uncomfortable episodes can be freely discussed. Such a climate can be most easily achieved in a peer group of doctors. This may be the partners in a practice or a small discussion group of colleagues from different practices.

The first example describes how one mistake was handled within a practice.

Drug allergy

At a practice meeting Dr Brown described a visit she had made to a Mrs Walmsley, who had developed a severe rash affecting the whole body. The patient was cross because she felt that the rash was similar to but worse than a previous drug reaction to a sulphonamide. Dr White had visited her three days before Dr Brown saw her and had prescribed co-trimoxazole for a urinary tract infection. The patient had assumed that the doctors knew that she was allergic to sulphonamides; only later did she realise that one of the ingredients of the prescribed antibiotic was a sulphonamide. Dr Brown and Dr White had already discussed the case before the meeting and had identified a number of points that they wished the partners to consider.

(1) The original call had been made at 9 pm on a Saturday evening. The symptoms had been present for two days but were increasingly severe and Mrs Walmsley complained of blood in the urine as well as frequency and dysuria. On the telephone Dr White ascertained that there had been no significant previous medical problem and did not pick up the

medical records before visiting the patient. On his way to Mrs Walmsley's house he received a potentially more serious call via his pager. As he was already nearly outside Mrs Walmsley's house he decided to see her before visiting the next patient.

(2) Dr White thought that he had asked Mrs Walmsley about possible allergies to antibiotics.

(3) Reviewing Mrs Walmsley's notes did not reveal any information about previous drug reactions on her summary card but continuation notes before 1980 had been removed by a previous doctor.

What would be the likely outcome of the practice meeting? The detailed discussions and possible changes in the arrangements for out of hours calls and in the data held in medical records can be left to the doctors concerned. The fact that the problem was discussed in a constructive and open fashion is of prime importance. Initially Dr Brown shared some of the patient's sense of outrage that this problem could have occurred. It would have been easy for the sake of superficial harmony within a practice for the episode to have been glossed over without resolving these feelings. The meeting allowed Dr White to understand the cumulative factors that contributed to the problem. As a result of the meeting not only Dr White but all the partners are likely to be more searching in future in eliciting possible drug allergies before prescribing.

What about the patient? After the practice meeting Dr White contacted Mrs Walmsley, who had now recovered both from the urinary tract infection and from the drug rash. She was invited to come and discuss her experience and at the consultation she was offered an apology and informed that the practice had discussed the problem and steps were being taken to avoid a recurrence. Mrs Walmsley was impressed by the serious way in which her problem had been taken up. On her part she would be certain to alert any future doctor about her drug allergy.

Wrong injection

A young principals' discussion group had been meeting each month for a year. As part of each meeting one doctor presented a recent clinical problem. On this occasion Dr Steven described her most recent immunisation clinic. By mistake she had omitted to give pertussis immunisation to a baby and had only given diphtheria and tetanus toxoids. Although the mistake was not of any immediate significance, Dr Steven was concerned that it had occurred and was in a dilemma about what she should do to rectify the mistake. Would informing the mother diminish her confidence in the practice? What would be the best way for the baby to catch up on pertussis immunisation?

The meeting, which had been in danger of sinking into torpor, suddenly became lively and animated. A consensus soon emerged about the practical steps to be taken. Most of the doctors felt that the mother should be informed straight away and offered a choice between an immediate pertussis immunisation for her child and a short wait until the next routine second immunisation, with a subsequent catching up for pertussis.

For Dr Steven the surprising aspect of the discussion was the interest shown by the other doctors in the precise arrangements for the immunisation clinic. Did she conduct the clinic alone? Who was responsible for recording the immunisations in the medical records and updating the practice and health board computer file on immunisations? How many children were seen at each session? From questions such as these it became clear that different practices organised clinics in very different ways. Given the different tasks Dr Steven was attempting to perform at the same time in her immunisation clinic it was felt that errors were inevitable.

Dr Steven's honesty in describing her error resulted in two tangible benefits. She returned to her own practice determined to make changes in the way her immunisation clinics were organised and serviced by practice staff. Armed with the constructive practical suggestions from her colleagues she was confident that changes could be implemented in her own practice. The discussion group itself also benefited from her initiative. A group that was in danger of disintegrating found new enthusiasm by being able to tackle a sensitive issue in an honest and supportive manner.

Neither the mother nor the baby was upset by the additional injection!

Neither of these two examples concerns life threatening problems. Fortunately such events are rare in general practice. The lessons that can be learnt from the recognition of clinical mistakes, however, do not depend on the seriousness of the clinical consequences. Indeed it may be easier to learn from less serious mistakes because blame and feelings of guilt are less likely to impede analysis of the factors involved than is the case for serious mistakes.

General practice is an operational specialty. Clinical mistakes are likely to involve organisational factors as well as pure clinical medicine. Indeed the identification of administrative errors is an excellent starting point for auditing practice organisation and will be considered further in the chapter on auditing the organisation.

Conclusion

Learning from the audit of clinically significant events is endless. The events that I have considered are just examples from the wide range of clinical material that is available. Further examples are considered in the chapter on auditing the organisation, because the audit of clinical events often reveals organisational as well as medical problems.

In this chapter I have tried to be positive and provocative about medical audit. The future of general practice will be bleak if audit is seen to be a mechanical process of data collection within a system that penalises deviations from the norm. I began the chapter by stating that the audit of clinically significant events raises more questions than answers. Audits should be cyclical activities in which structured inquiry leads to a deeper understanding of the processes of care and to the formulation of better questions and better ways of collecting information. Research and audit are sometimes considered to be separate activities, but good audit projects lead to questions that can be researched and are of general relevance.

1 New Leeuwenhorst Group. *Quality improvement by quality assessment—a first statement*. Amsterdam: Huisarten Instituut Vinje Universiteit Amsterdam, 1986.
2 Pendleton D (ed). *The consultation: an approach to learning and teaching*. Oxford: Oxford University Press, 1984.
3 Byrne P, Long BEL. *Doctors talking to patients*. London: Royal College of General Practitioners, 1976.
4 Stott N, Davis RH. The exceptional potential in each primary care consultant. *J R Coll Gen Pract* 1979;**29**:201–5.

Further reading
Anonymous. Critical questions; critical incidents; critical answers. *Lancet* 1988;i: 1373–4.
Newble DI. The critical incident technique: a new approach to the assessment of clinical performance. *Medical Education* 1983:**167**;401–30.

Auditing the organisation

GRAHAM BUCKLEY

Introduction

The overall aims of general practice are to maintain the health of the practice population and meet the perceived health needs of patients in a manner that is acceptable to them. No statement of the aims of general practice will meet with universal approval. Put in these terms, however, general practice encompasses a range of services broader than those traditionally provided. Health promotion and the prevention of disease have been accepted by the profession, by the government, and increasingly by patients as integral parts of general practice. The benefits of programmes of disease prevention and health promotion are in the main cherished hopes rather than proven facts. Nevertheless, there is no doubt that general practitioners need to provide a proactive service as well as a reactive one. These new responsibilities add enormously to the organisational requirements of a practice. Providing a proactive service in which children and adults are offered immunisations, screening, and health checks requires not only a major expansion in administrative resources but will probably also require members of the practice team, especially the doctors, to change their attitudes.

The green and white papers on the future of primary care in the health service give a high priority to the development of preventive care. This has been translated in the new contractual requirements for general practitioners as meaning the need to document different types of preventive and health promotional work carried out within the practice if payment is to be received. The new contractual requirements will test all practice organisations not only in providing the services but also in demonstrating that the work has been done.

Some practices are keen to take on the additional managerial responsibilities of operating a practice budget. Whatever the political and ethical issues involved the opportunity to operate practice budgets has only been granted because of the confidence the government has in the ability of some general practitioners to manage their practices efficiently and effectively.

General practice can be considered as a service industry. In an increasingly consumerist society practices are likely to be judged by patients by the criteria that apply to other services. Hairdressers and garages are judged on the basis of geographical convenience, ease of access, and the welcome provided by reception staff, as well as the quality of the service performed. Patients have to assume the technical competence of a general practitioner and thus have to rely on other aspects of a practice in forming a judgment.

We may feel uncomfortable at being judged by the same criteria as commercial services, but the government is keen to promote competition between practices. It is the organisational aspects of the practice that are likely to be crucial in attracting new patients. Restrictions on advertising by doctors are being relaxed and practices are now obliged to provide practice leaflets that describe the range of services offered by the practice.

Doctors, patients, and the government each have standards and criteria by which they form judgments about a practice. From the patient's point of view general practice should be easily *accessible* and services should be provided in an *acceptable* way. The government and doctors share a desire for practices to be *efficient* in the use of limited resources. The government will be particularly concerned with the efficient use of money; doctors will possibly be more concerned with the efficient use of time and personnel.

Patients, doctors, and the government all wish general practice to be *effective*. Much of this book concerns the auditing of clinical activities as a means of helping general practitioners to become more effective in their clinical work. Throughout the whole of clinical medicine it is difficult to find good criteria for judging effectiveness. For the most part it is necessary to look at the processes of care rather than the outcome. This is equally true for practice organisation. Management, like medicine, is an inexact science and largely concerns human relationships. No one type of practice organisation is ideal. Practices vary according to the strengths and weaknesses of their own personnel and according to the other health care resources available in the locality.

Before looking at ways of auditing the accessibility, acceptability, efficiency, and effectiveness of the practice it is worth while defining the context in which individual items of service are provided. This means looking at the overall management style of the practice and the overall workload.

Management styles

Unless the basic management style of the practice is understood barriers to change may frustrate useful initiatives. Many doctors remain sceptical about the need to develop managerial skills. Their scepticism is understandable. Doctors have lengthy training to develop their clinical skills but formal training in management remains a rarity for them. The academic base of management is founded in sociology and psychology and doctors reading the standard textbooks may be deterred by the language.

Likert[1] has described four basic styles of organisation: authoritative exploitative; authoritative benign; consultative; and participative. An examination of recent decisions within a practice will reveal the type of management that is operating—for example, the introduction of late night surgery sessions one evening a week. The way in which such a change is initiated, agreed, and implemented indicates the management style. It is likely that many practices will oscillate between an authoritative benign style of management and a consultative one, depending on the particular management decisions being considered. On financial matters general practitioners may wish to reserve to themselves all discussion and decision making. In other aspects of practice organisation doctors will wish to consult other members of the primary health care team and sometimes encourage them to participate in making decisions.

The structure of organisation within a practice is therefore complex: it combines elements of hierarchy, matrix, and team relationships. This complexity reflects the different ways in which practice members are employed: independent contractor doctors employing secretarial staff and practice nurses working with district nurses and health visitors who are employed by the health authority. This complexity has encouraged the adoption in primary health care of dynamic concepts of organisation, as in systems theory. The approach is in tune with medical audit because it concentrates on measuring the input and output of a system with feedback as the mechanism for achieving a dynamic equilibrium. Stripped of its jargon this approach encourages a primary health care team to define what it is trying to achieve; to make the best possible use of the available physical and human resources; to measure the outcome of care; and to use this information to redefine the original tasks. Books and videos for further study of this subject are given at the end of the chapter.

In a small organisation like a general practice it is likely that informal discussions are at least as influential as overt formal methods. Particular styles of organisation are of no intrinsic merit but are to be judged by their effectiveness. By developing an understanding of the way in which the organisation functions the possibility for implementing change is enhanced. It is futile to audit specific aspects of the practice if change cannot be implemented.

Meetings

Practice meetings are essential for the organisation to function. Without regular meetings planning new services and auditing existing activities are impossible. Meetings require careful planning if they are to be effective. Few general practitioners enjoy meetings about practice organisation. Escape from the hierarchical structure and bureaucracy of hospital medicine may be among the motivating factors for doctors choosing general practice as a career. General practice, however, is now a complex activity requiring sophisticated organisation. Meetings can be made enjoyable as well as effective if their purpose is explicit, if discussion is kept to the point, and if note is taken of decisions reached.

Meetings themselves can be audited. Answers to the following questions will indicate whether a meeting has a chance of being successful.

- Are the aims of the meeting clearly understood by the participants? If the aims have not been made clear by circulating relevant papers and an agenda before the meeting then clarifying the aims should be the first item for discussion.
- Have all the relevant people within the practice been notified and invited?
- Are all the agenda items essential and is enough time available to get through the agenda?

- Can the chairperson of the meeting keep the discussion relevant to the points to be discussed?
- Is a note made of the decisions reached at the meeting? Is it clear who is to take responsibility for acting upon these decisions?

In the video *Meetings, Bloody Meetings*[2] John Cleese shows how it is possible to destroy effective communication. Within all organisations there is a danger that meetings may become an end in themselves. They are expensive in terms of staff time and the questions listed above will help to determine whether some meetings are required at all. Nevertheless, some regular meetings are required within a practice. A short meeting in which all members of the practice participate should be held each week as a clearing house for information. These meetings need only take a quarter of an hour but are essential in providing everyone in the practice with the opportunity of raising issues as well as of exchanging information. Important issues may then need to be explored in more detail by the people directly concerned. It is common for the partners in a practice to meet monthly to review the performance of the practice. Increasingly practice managers are taking an active part in these doctors' meetings and will contribute in providing information from audits of the organisation on which decisions about possible changes will be made.

Workload

The chapter on practice reports describes the ways in which practice workload data can be gathered and presented. It is helpful to translate the yearly rates and totals present in the practice report into numbers that describe average working days and working weeks. It is then possible to see whether present arrangements are adequate or are under strain.

Six thousand consultations a year would place a doctor in the lower half of the range for the United Kingdom. In a four partner practice this would mean that each week an average of 480 appointments would need to be provided for patients. (This calculation assumes a 50 week year to take into account public holidays and to make the arithmetic simpler) Although there is considerable day to day fluctuation in the number of people seen in a general practice, there is little variation from week to week even in times of influenza epidemics because most of the fluctuation is in the number of home visits requested. Day to day variation in appointments is partly a function of practice arrangements (traditionally few appointments are provided on a Wednesday) and partly a function of differences in demand from the patients, with more requests made on a Monday.

In spite of information on workload being readily available, many practices still choose to provide surgery sessions on the basis of tradition rather than planning. If practices only offer enough appointments each week to cope with average demand then it is inevitable that minor fluctuations in demand will create a recurrent strain on the system, with receptionists having to fit in extra patients as best they can and with general practitioners extending their consulting sessions in an unpredictable and consequently stressful fashion.

In the example above if one doctor is on holiday the remaining three will each need to see an extra 40 patients during the week—that is, an extra eight patients per doctor per day. For each day of the partner's holiday the remaining partners should therefore assume that they will need to increase their consulting time by approximately one and half hours. This seems so simple and yet many practices just muddle through with consequent increased stress for patients, receptionists, and doctors.

Other major elements of workload from the point of view of the doctor are home visits, telephone consultations, writing letters and reports, and administration. Each of these activities is quantifiable and should be included in the planning of a working week.

Table 1 shows the timetable of Dr A, a doctor in the practice described above. He provides 116 appointments a week, eight unbooked consultations on a Friday, and the possibility of extending the consultation session on three afternoons a week.

It is clear that Doctor A provides just enough appointments to cope with average demand while giving time on Tuesday mornings and Thursday afternoons for administrative tasks. In the absence of one doctor from the practice these sessions would be eroded by the need to provide more consulting time.

This analysis of the ways in which the practice meets anticipated workload is a necessary part of medical audit. It enables data collected from surveys of workload to be interpreted in the appropriate context and thus helps to suggest solutions to the organisational problems that are identified.

Similar planning for other members of the primary health care

TABLE 1—Dr A's timetable

	Monday	Tuesday	Wednesday	Thursday	Friday
8.30	Consulting (10)	Duty doctor	Consulting (8)	Practice meeting	Consulting (10)
9.30					
10.30				Consulting (8)	
11.30	Consulting (8)	For home visits	Child surveillance clinic	Consulting (6)	Consulting (8)
12.30	Home visits				
13.30	Lunch meeting	Consulting (10)	Chronic visits + duty doctor for afternoon visits	Administration	
14.30	Antenatal clinic				Consulting (10)
15.30					
16.30	Consulting (12)	Consulting (8)	Consulting (10)	Consulting (8)	Unbooked consulting
17.30					
18.30					
Extension number	Yes	No	Yes	Yes

Figures in parentheses show the number of appointment slots at intervals of seven minutes.

team can take place if basic information about workload is available. For example, it can be calculated for the secretarial and reception staff that for each consultation with the doctor or practice nurse at least two contacts are made with the reception staff: one to make the appointment and one to report on arrival at the practice premises. In addition to these contacts there are requests for repeat prescriptions and results of investigations. If we take the example of the four partner practice already described the number of contacts with the secretarial and reception staff will approach 2000 a week. If there are four full time secretary receptionists each will have approximately 100 contacts with patients each day. Such contacts are only part of their duties. Secretary receptionists are expected to type letters and medical reports; maintain practice information systems with data on immunisations, cervical smears, morbidity, etc; send claim forms to the health authority for item of service payments; file information and records; and look out records for consultation sessions and replace them at the end of the day.

From the above comments about general practice workload it can be seen that it is a high volume operation in which human interactions are measured each day in tens and hundreds. General practice is about people and long term relationships. Given the high level of activity it would be remarkable if all the interactions were uniformly successful. Some exchanges between doctors, receptionists, nurses, and patients will be less than perfect, and meeting all the expressed health care wants of patients is impossible. The motive underlying medical audit is the recognition that there are always opportunities to improve the services provided by a practice. Positive motivation towards undertaking medical audit is likely to result from a balance of internal and external factors. Internal motivation flows from the spirit of inquiry that should be fostered in educational activity for *all* members of the primary health care team. This internal motivation is enhanced by the successful outcome of an audit project and the personal satisfaction that comes from the knowledge of doing one's work well.

Access

Good access is basic to any service. Delay before being able to see a doctor is a commonly heard criticism of general practice. There are several aspects to access: geographical, physical, personal, and psychological. It is of no advantage to the patient to be seen at the time and place of his or her choosing if the doctor is exhausted after a night on duty and is unable to function effectively. Access is always likely to be a compromise between the wishes of the patients and the resources of the practice. In North America walk in health shops provide easy access but low continuity of care. General practices in the United Kingdom provide patients with the opportunity for continuity of care and many people seem to value this, particularly older patients. Cultural differences between countries influence expectations about the accessibility of doctors. Even within the United Kingdom the number of night visits carried out by general practitioners varies enormously. It is therefore sensible for practices to adapt their patterns of work to local needs. General practitioners have been criticised for using deputising services for night and weekend cover but this may be a sensible policy for an inner city practice attempting to cope with a high level of demand during the day. Audit encourages us to develop practice policies on access that are based on evidence rather than prejudice. Access is crucial in determining how a practice is viewed by its patients. It makes sense to seek the views of patients when developing practice policies about access.

Appointment systems

Most practices now run some form of appointment system. The advantage of such a system is that it spreads the work evenly throughout the week and minimises the time that patients have to spend in the waiting room. Before auditing the system the practice should try to establish such standard rules as:

- Patients with urgent problems (as perceived by them) should be offered same day appointments
- All patients should be offered an appointment within 24 hours
- All patients should be offered an appointment with their personal doctor within 72 hours.

As well as being useful in the audit of an appointment system these rules help reception staff to make appointments and inform doctors when extra consulting time is needed.

The simplest way to audit an appointments system is to examine the appointment book in the early afternoon. If all appointments for the same day are already taken up and half the next day appointments are also booked then receptionists will have great difficulty meeting the above standards. Regular monitoring of the available same day and next day appointments will produce data that may reveal a regular pattern and suggest changes that could be made; for example, monitoring the appointment book each day at 2 pm in the four partner practice previously described gave the results shown in table 2.

At the audit meeting at which these results were discussed the receptionist confirmed that there had been difficulty in providing appointments for patients who contacted the surgery on Monday morning and afternoon. For some of the doctors the first available appointment was on Wednesday morning. The figures for the practice suggested two related problems. Firstly, 40 out of the 100 Monday appointments had already been booked by the end of the previous week; secondly, the demand for appointments on a

TABLE 2—Results of monitoring the appointment book in a four partner practice at 2 pm each day

	Appointments originally available	Same day appointments available	Next day appointments available
Monday	100	0	40
Tuesday	100	2	40
Wednesday	80	20	80
Thursday	100	40	60
Friday	100	30	60*

* Monday.

Monday exceeds supply and creates a cascade effect on the following days of the week. This effect lasts until Wednesday afternoon. On Thursday a number of appointments remain unbooked. The conclusion was that the practice was providing enough appointments but that they were poorly distributed. It was decided that a new policy could be created on the following lines:

- Returning patients would be dissuaded from prebooking on a Monday.
- More appointments would be provided on Mondays at the expense of Thursday appointments.

A more sophisticated but more time consuming audit would be to construct a scoring sheet (table 3) for receptionists to complete when making appointments for patients.

TABLE 3—Sheet for receptionists to complete on Mondays on asking patients "When would you like an appointment?"

Patient	Today	Tomorrow	Later	Delay between preferred and offered appointment times	Appointment with own doctor
1		1		1	
2	1			0	
3			1	1	1
4		1		0	
5			1	1	1
6	1			0	1

This type of audit gives detailed information about patterns of demand for appointments and starts to explore the delicate subject of the availability of different doctors within the practice.

Work sharing between doctors in a partnership is a regular source of conflict, but the subject tends to be avoided at practice meetings by discussion of less sensitive topics. This is unfortunate because, if tackled in a constructive fashion, it can lead to much better relationships between partners, better job satisfaction for doctors, and a better service for patients. Drawing up equal personal lists of patients is one way of ensuring equity in workload within a practice. Creating personal lists also clarifies clinical responsibility for the patient.

In the next section in this chapter we look at another aspect of each doctor's performance.

Delay in the waiting room

Receptionists will be aware of the irritation felt by patients who have to wait a long time in the waiting room before seeing the doctor. One of the aims of an appointment system is to minimise the time patients have to spend in the waiting room. These times can be measured by the receptionist noting the time of arrival, time of appointment, and time called in to see the doctor for each patient; but a more useful audit involves the general practitioner noting the time of the start and the end of consultations. Figure 1 shows the way in which the times can be plotted to show the progress of consultations in each session. If this analysis is repeated for a number of sessions it gives information in the following areas:

(1) Average length of consultations. In the example the average length of a consultation is 9.5 minutes for a series of appointments that are booked at 7.5 minutes intervals.

(2) Average waiting time. In the example the average waiting time from arrival of the patient was 16 minutes and from the time of the appointment was 13 minutes.

Telephone access

A common complaint is the difficulty of contacting the practice by telephone. The practice may not be aware of this because, obviously, only calls that get through are responded to. General practitioners know how frustrating it is to be unable to get through on the telephone to hospital departments. Hospital colleagues and

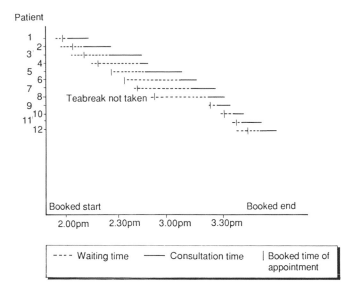

FIGURE 1—Plot showing progress of consultations in an afternoon surgery. (Courtesy of Professor JGR Howie.)

patients share the same frustrations if they are unable to get through to the practice.

At an audit meeting members of the practice team could be asked to express their concern about the telephone system and the accessibility of doctors on the telephone. The first concern is likely to be about the inability of the system to cope with calls at peak times.

A standard in this area is easy to state but difficult to assess: *it should be possible to contact a practice by telephone without delay at all times of day.*

With some modern switchboards it is possible to monitor whether all lines are in use. Without this facility the telephonist would have to monitor incoming calls over selected periods and also ask callers if they have had difficulty in contacting the practice. Peak demand is likely to be during the first two hours of the morning. Monitoring this period would give an indication of whether the telephone system was adequate. Even if the practice does have an adequate number of telephone lines the operator may be so busy at times of peak demand that he or she cannot respond immediately to a new call. Transfer of calls within the practice may

155

be inefficient. With the provision of some objective information the discussions at the next practice audit meeting might lead to the creation of new practice policies as in the following:

- Outgoing calls for the practice should, whenever possible, be made in the afternoon. This helps to keep lines free in the mornings for incoming calls
- To make it easier to find them staff should make use of diversion facilities on internal phones to make their location easier
- Patients should be encouraged to phone only in the afternoon for results of investigations etc.

Such a policy has several advantages. It reduces the demand on the telephone system in the mornings. Letters and reports are likely to be processed within the morning and the results made available by the afternoon. Requests for information can be handled more efficiently if they are concentrated within a limited period.

Availability of doctor on the telephone

At the audit meeting doctors may complain about frequent interruptions during consultations; receptionists may say that because patients cannot contact doctors on the telephone they put in requests for home visits. Without information it may not be possible to formulate a sensible practice policy; but an audit can solve that problem.

Receptionists should log the requests patients make to speak to the doctor on the telephone. A suitable form for the purpose is shown in table 4.

The doctors should simply make a note of all telephone calls they receive when they are seeing patients in their consulting rooms. From the information gained from this simple audit the practice might agree to adopt the following policy:

TABLE 4—Availability of doctor on the telephone

	Requests to speak to doctor	Doctor unavailable	Call put through	Request dealt with by the secretary
Monday	******	**	*	***
Tuesday				
Wednesday				
Thursday				
Friday				

- The practice to inform patients that the best time to phone if they wish to speak directly to the doctor is between 3 pm and 4 pm.
- If patients phone at other times with requests that are not urgent they are to be asked to leave a telephone number or phone again between 3 pm and 4 pm.

It may, however, be impossible to agree a policy that will operate throughout the practice because the doctors may have different styles of consulting and different outside commitments; some of the partners may wish to be available during normal consulting sessions and others may wish to be protected from all but urgent calls. At least the audit meeting can make these differences clear so that receptionists have a chance of dealing with telephone calls in a reasonable way.

Acceptability

If a practice and its services are reasonably accessible the next major point to be considered is whether the practice meets the expectations of its registered patients.

Public opinion surveys show that people are critical about delays in being seen by general practitioners and about hurried consultations. When asked about their own doctor, however, people are much more positive and will make excuses for perceived deficiencies. There are strong emotional factors that tend to encourage positive comments by patients about their own family doctor. It may be too disquieting for individuals to harbour criticisms about a personal service that may have to be relied on in a time of crisis. In addition many patients have known their own doctor for many years and, as in all long term relationships, personal foibles become accepted and tolerated. Patients may fear that the voicing of criticisms may prejudice the doctor against them in future consultations. It is therefore difficult to extract critical comments about a practice directly from patients. Any criticisms that are voiced should be carefully considered. Spontaneous criticisms are unusual events but can raise issues that have general importance for the practice organisation.

Complaints

Does the practice have a clear policy on how complaints should be handled? If not there is the risk of compounding a complaint by giving an insensitive response. Even if complaints are ill founded they may indicate a failure in the organisation because patients have not been adequately informed about practice policies. All members of the practice are likely to receive complaints; equally, they are likely to have complaints made about them. It is therefore vital that all staff should know how to cope with complaints and what patients' rights are. The issues raised by the complaint should certainly be reviewed. But it may be worth while to examine also the way in which it was handled. To this end the following questions may be relevant.

- Was the patient given the opportunity and time to express the complaint fully?
- Was the patient offered a quiet room to discuss the complaint or was his or her only alternative a harassed exchange with the receptionist in a busy waiting room?
- Was the patient given a chance to discuss the complaint with the relevant person in authority—for example, was he or she offered an interview with the doctor or the practice manager?
- Was the patient informed of the ways in which formal complaints can be dealt with?

For complaints about failures in practice organisation a formal complaint should normally be sent to the administrator of the family practitioner committee.

From the point of view of audit, whatever the outcome of the complaint itself—and in the main patients are content with a full discussion and the knowledge that the complaint is being taken seriously—the practice can make use of the episode to look at practice organisation. The following examples illustrate this point.

Rude receptionist

A patient complained that the receptionist was rude and abrupt on the telephone when he asked for the result of a blood test. The complaint was handled in the way outlined above and after an interview with his own general practitioner the patient decided not to take the matter further. A subsequent discussion between the receptionist, the practice manager, and the doctor revealed two problems:

(1) The lack of a clear policy about which investigation results may be given to patients over the telephone.
(2) The receptionist concerned felt under a lot of pressure as she was covering for a colleague who was absent.

It is easier to solve the first problem than the second. A new policy on procedure can be created whereby doctors indicate on the report slips whether or not the information can be given over the telephone to patients.

Alleviating stress within a practice is an important but endless task. Some members of staff cope better than others with enforced changes in workload brought about by increased patient demand or the unexpected absence of colleagues. Complaints may indicate that stress has reached an unacceptable level and staff morale is deteriorating. Recognising these problems is the first step towards dealing with them. This aspect of audit is considered later in this chapter under the heading "Staff."

Missed call

A patient phoned at 4 pm to complain that although he had got in touch with the surgery at 10 am to ask for a home visit, the doctor had not yet arrived. His medical condition had improved but he still wanted the doctor to visit and thought that the delay was unreasonable. The cause of the delay was soon identified. The paper slip containing details of the request had gone astray and the duty doctor did not know about the call. The duplicate copy of the form confirmed that the request was made. The doctor visited the patient and after finding that there was no serious medical problem explained the mistake and promised to look into the arrangements for receiving requests.

At the subsequent audit meeting a number of people voiced anxieties about the risk of losing house visit slips and it was agreed that a new system should be introduced. After consultation with all members of staff it was agreed to have a permanent register of home visit requests, using a book that permits copies of details to be produced automatically.

As well as being less risky, the new method makes it easier to collect data on the number and timing of home visits. This not only assists in the production of the annual report of the practice but may also indicate when resources for home visits are inadequate.

Near misses

It is not necessary to wait until the disaster happens or the complaint is made before using errors as the starting point for audit. The staff may be aware of potential errors even if these are not noticed by patients. For example, an error in a repeat prescription may be spotted by the medical secretary before it is issued to the patient or by the pharmacist before it is dispensed—pyridostigmine instead of pyridoxine; carbimazole instead of carbamazepine. Misfiling of information is possible if fathers and sons or mothers and daughters share the same names. This can create havoc medically and socially—for example, by the misfiling of the daughter's pregnancy test in the mother's notes.

The practice can have a near miss book in which members of the practice can record near misses in which they have been personally involved. The book can then be the starting point for audit meeting discussions about practice organisation.

Patient satisfaction

I have already suggested that it is difficult to elicit critical comments directly from patients about a practice. Constructive criticism is more likely if the questioning comes from respected independent agencies such as the Community Health Council or a team of research workers. Even these agencies tend to receive positive views about services. Patients tend to accept the particular style of service provided by their own practice. There are, however, some criticisms of general practice that do seem to be widespread: the reluctance of doctors to carry out home visits; the difficulty in seeing one's own doctor; the rigidity of appointment systems; receptionists who act as barriers between patients and doctors; and consultations considered as too hurried.

Patient participation groups are one mechanism for ascertaining the views of patients. The existence of such a group locally may allow patients' views in general to be channelled back to the practice. An outward looking practice will encourage members of staff to participate in local community activities. This is not only of direct benefit to the community but is also a means of discovering whether the practice is meeting the needs of the community that it serves.

If major changes in practice organisation are contemplated—for example, the introduction of a health promotion clinic for men—then a survey of the relevant patient group is worth while. In designing a questionnaire it is important that the questions should be clear, unambiguous, and capable of interpretation. In the box on page 161 is an example of how such a questionnaire might be set out. Patients attending the surgery may constitute the sample.

Although these patients are not truly representative of the total practice population, it is the simplest and cheapest way of obtaining the views of a large number of patients. The space for comments at the bottom of the questionnaire are likely to range from the rude to the complimentary but may indicate aspects of practice organisation that could be suitable for audit.

THE PRACTICE PLANS TO HOLD A WELL MAN CLINIC

This will provide a health check every two years for men between 25 and 60 and will offer advice on how to improve fitness.

Are you interested in attending the clinic?

YES ☐   NO ☐   Please tick

We plan to hold the clinic on either Wednesday afternoon or Thursday evening. Please indicate which time you would prefer.

Wednesday afternoon (2–4 pm) ☐
Thursday evening (6–8 pm)   ☐   Please tick

We are interested to have feedback about the services we provide. Please use the space below for any comments you wish to make about the practice.

....

....

....

....

As family doctors we share a belief that general practice is the best way of providing primary medical care. It is a belief which needs a stream of research evidence to sustain it. Recent government legislation keeps general practice at the centre of the National Health Service by preserving the referral system to specialists. This privileged position carries with it heavy responsibilities, one of which is the need to ensure that people want what we provide.

Effectiveness and efficiency

Clinical effectiveness and efficiency are covered in other chapters of this book. Here I shall be considering the operational aspects of clinical management. The continuing health of many people depends on effective practice administration more than the clinical acumen of doctors. The example I shall use is repeat prescriptions. It is also possible to look at immunisation programmes, cervical smears, uptake rates, and case screening in the elderly.

Repeat prescriptions

A repeat prescription service is a relatively recent development in general practice. Its growth matches the extraordinary growth in the number and potency of drugs that the pharmaceutical industry has developed in the past 30 years. Nevertheless, some practices only issue prescriptions at face to face consultations and prescribe enough drugs to last for three months for patients with chronic health problems such as hypertension.

Assuming that the practice does have a repeat prescription system the following questions will be addressed in the audit of the system.

- Who is eligible for a repeat prescription? How is the information entered in the system? What are the patients' expectations of the system?
- How is a request handled?
- How is the accuracy of the prescription checked?
- Are patients regularly reviewed? Is the need for repeat prescriptions monitored?
- How much time does the practice spend on this service?

Repeat prescription modules are an important feature of the computer software packages that are on offer to general practitioners. In assessing these packages it is useful for practices to consider how manual systems can be audited and therefore the features that a computerised system should include.

The following standards might be adopted for auditing repeat prescribing.

- Eligibility for repeat prescriptions clearly stated within the medical records
- Names, quantities, and instructions for use of drugs clearly stated and understood by staff and patients
- Date of last prescription stated
- Date of last and next review of medications known and stated
- Requests for repeat prescriptions processed within 24 hours.

The practical steps for auditing the repeat prescriptions system are straightforward. A list of people receiving repeat prescriptions can be generated by logging them as they request prescriptions during one month. Most people receiving repeat prescriptions will be included. The total number will indicate the level of repeat prescribing and permit comparisons with data from other practices. Many of the patients on repeat prescriptions require active monitoring—for example, diabetic patients and those receiving thyroxin diuretics or anticonvulsants. An examination of the records of these patients will give information about when they were last seen. Surveys have indicated some disappointing levels of surveillance; occasionally several years elapse before people taking digoxin or thyroxine are reviewed.

Computer systems have an inbuilt recall system incorporated into repeat prescribing packages. These systems, however, can be overridden and it is still worth while checking in the patients' records to see whether reviews are in fact taking place.

A 24 hour processing time is a common feature of a repeat prescribing system, but it is unnecessary. Producing prescriptions in anticipation of demand is possible provided that the information system is accurate. Patients can then request to receive prescriptions as a one stop procedure. Preproduction of repeat prescriptions can be done in a calm, systematic fashion that is likely to improve arrangements for monitoring the drugs and reviewing the patients' need for them.

Staff

Efficient and effective practice organisation requires the active participation of all staff. Teamwork has become a hackneyed term of exhortation rather than a realistic description of the way in which primary health care services are organised. Structural differences in the employment of district nurses, health visitors, and general practitioners impede full teamwork. In general practice teamwork is essential. Medical secretaries and receptionists have been almost invisible in much of the literature about primary care and their essential contribution has been overlooked.

The nature of general practice requires staff to be more than just competent at administrative tasks. It requires flexibility, commitment, and resourcefulness. Patients expect warmth with their prescriptions and interest with their appointments.

It is possible to audit elements of the work of secretaries and receptionists but it would be foolhardy to do so without full participation and active interest from the staff. Audit can and should become a method of increasing job satisfaction rather than being perceived as a threat. Audit should therefore arise out of discussions about concerns that the staff raise.

As general practice becomes more sophisticated in its organisation more and more is expected of the administrative staff. It is rare for any activities to cease when new tasks are identified. If secretarial staff believe that the doctors are listening to their concerns and have an understanding of the administrative workload this makes a good basis for integrating audit into practice organisation. One simple audit that could improve the efficiency of the practice would be to measure the time taken to locate files in preparation for a consultation session. Searching for missing files is likely to make the task take considerably longer than it should, and the solution to this problem is likely to lie in the hands of the doctors rather than the secretaries. With the confidence gained from participating in audit projects receptionists may be willing to look at their own interviewing skills through role play or, with the permission of patients, video recording interviews at the reception desk.

Staff appraisal

The requirement for practices to produce annual reports could result in a boring data collection exercise. Dr Pringle demonstrates (pages 196–223) how the production of these reports can be a stimulating and challenging activity that encourages practices to define what they are trying to achieve and how best to do it. This concept applies to people as well as to practice activities. Studies in job satisfaction and achievement in a number of different settings have demonstrated that, once basic financial requirements are satisfied, job satisfaction comes from knowing that one's work is valued by one's peers and those in authority. Personal feedback in the form of annual appraisals could become part of the audit of the practice. This applies to doctors just as much as to secretarial staff. Setting targets for the coming year and reviewing whether previous targets have been met are useful in both organisational and personal terms.

Buildings and equipment

The physical surroundings and facilities of a practice may appear to be so self evident that they do not lend themselves to an audit project. Deficiencies in the number of rooms or space for records or even in the integrity of the roof may be all too obvious. It is important, however, for premises to be acceptable to patients, to be tolerable for staff, and to *function* effectively. One test of function is to try to get into the practice premises in a wheelchair. Even ground floor premises may be inaccessible because of narrow doors, doorsteps, and high reception counters.

Although it is easy to list the equipment held within the practice its use still needs to be audited. One way of doing this is to have a test run of a cardiac arrest. This will reveal: (*a*) if reception staff know how to contact doctors in an emergency; (*b*) if everybody knows where the emergency equipment is kept; and (*c*) if the nurses and doctors know how to use the equipment.

Basic cardiopulmonary resuscitation is a simple skill that anyone can learn in a short time. The figures for successful resuscitation will only increase when large numbers of the general public are able to provide mouth to mouth breathing and external cardiac massage. There is a case for all who are involved in health care to be able to undertake basic resuscitation. The mannikins that are now available make it possible to test this skill in a simple and objective way.

Records

I have left audit of patient records to the end of this chapter. They are so important, and so easy to audit, that it is easy for attention to be focused on this aspect of practice organisation to the detriment of other important areas. There is also a danger that records may be seen as ends in themselves rather than as tools in improving patient care. The medical record now includes information held in computers as well as the written individual record. Computer held information is already accessible to patients, and it is only a matter of time before written records are made generally available to patients. A number of practices already routinely give patients their own records. This can be seen as one form of audit and is effective in revealing errors about previous medical events. More conventional practices will establish standards that they wish to achieve. The following checklist is derived from the guidelines published by the Joint Higher Training Committee for General Practice for teaching practices.

- Summary of health problems
- Letters in chronological order
- Legible clinical notes
- Up to date medicine list
- Relevant basic data: immunisation status, date of cervical smear, weight and height, date of last blood pressure measurement, functional assessment of older patients.

If medical records meet the above criteria they will be more than an effective aide mémoire: they will also help doctors reach diagnoses and provide a basis for health promotion. Although it is easy to scrutinise a random sample of records, it is sometimes more useful to look at selected age groups. For this an age/sex register is needed. To fulfil the requirements of the new contract it is important for the manual records to be backed up by a computer information system.

It is likely that a first audit of the medical records will reveal deficiencies: perhaps only half of the records have a summary of health problems and in three quarters the basic data may be incomplete. The practice can then set targets to be achieved within a specified period; a repeat audit will reveal whether these targets have been reached.

Conclusion

Change in general practice is normal, but it is now taking place at a breathtaking speed. Without efficient organisation general practitioners will not be able to cope with the increasing responsibilities and requirements of their new contract.

Auditing the organisation should not become another bureaucratic burden. Instead it should be a process of critical inquiry that can enliven even routine tasks and give proper prominence to previously neglected areas such as reception work. The best possible outcome of an audit into an aspect of organisation is that the practice team should look forward to its next audit project.

1 Likert R. *New patterns of management*. New York: McGraw-Hill, 1961.
2 Cleese, John. *Meetings, bloody meetings*. London: Video Arts Ltd, 1988

Further reading and viewing

Cartwright A, Anderson R. *General practice revisited*. London: Tavistock, 1981. (A monograph giving the patient's perspective of general practice.)

Jones RVH *et al. Running a practice*. London: Croom Helm, 1985. (A practical book that tackles the basic aspects of practice organisation.)

Pritchard P, Low K, Whalen M. *Management in general practice*. Oxford: Oxford University Press, 1986. (An excellent book dealing with the aims, tasks, and skills of general practice.)

Huntingdon J, Irvine S (for the MSD Foundation). *Management in practice*. London: Royal College of General Practitioners, 1985. (Video and course books, particularly useful for stimulating discussion and debate within a practice.)

Royal College of General Practitioners. *If only I had the time*. London: Royal College of General Practitioners, 1989. (Distance learning package.)

Statistical issues in medical audit

IAN RUSSELL, DAPHNE RUSSELL

In this chapter, we show how statistical principles can help in the conduct and then the interpretation of an audit. To set this discussion in context we first identify some of the differences and similarities between medical audit and medical research—the activity within medicine with which the application of statistical principles is traditionally associated.

Audit and research: differences and similarities

Most statistical advice to doctors in lectures and textbooks is directed towards the doctor doing research. Much of this also applies to audit, but there are at least three important differences.

Firstly, the researcher, even if the data came from only a few practices (or even one!), is interested in drawing inferences about a general population of patients, doctors, or practices; he or she will usually concentrate on a small subset of practice activities. In contrast, an audit seeks to draw inferences about only one doctor or practice, but will aim (eventually) to cover a representative selection of practice activities.

Secondly, in audit a given practice's results are compared with a predetermined standard so that the appropriate statistical procedure is a hypothesis test answering the question, "Are we falling significantly short of the standard?" Although hypothesis tests are used in research, the researcher is more often interested in estimation—for example, by confidence intervals.

Thirdly, most researchers either compare two or more samples or investigate the relationship between many variables. In audit a single sample is compared with a standard, one variable at a time.

168

Despite these differences the doctor undertaking audit needs to abide by most of the basic principles of research: precision in defining objectives and procedures; careful planning so that the data he or she needs are available, unbiased, and reliable; rigorous sampling methods and statistical analysis; and clear presentation of results and conclusions.

Sampling and bias

Enumerate or sample?

When comparing practice performance with a specified standard one may either *enumerate* all relevant patients within the practice or sample only some of the relevant patients and infer from them the overall practice performance.

Enumeration should be used where the standard of interest refers to routine and readily available statistics, often already compiled for another purpose. Examples in the final chapter in this book include practice immunisation rates (table 18, page 211) and cervical smear uptake (table 20, page 211); although numbers are large and sampling would give perfectly adequate estimates of the rates, it is as easy (or easier) to count all patients, provided that the data needed are already in the practice computer. As the information held on practice computers becomes more sophisticated and detailed the range of topics for which enumeration is feasible will increase. Enumeration will also be necessary if the event of interest is so rare that all relevant patients need to be examined.

EXAMPLE 1—In any one year there will be relatively few cancer deaths in a single practice (see, for example, table 17, page 210). If you want to compare your terminal care with an agreed protocol you should use all such patients even if extra work is required for the comparison.

Sampling, however, is recommended whenever a detailed analysis of the whole practice or a large subgroup of patients, consultations, or activities is required. Limiting audit to areas that can easily be enumerated is too restrictive.

The detailed analysis may be done retrospectively by examining existing records or prospectively by using an extra recording sheet for the sampled patients or consultations to provide more detail than would otherwise be available. An example of retrospective analysis is given in table 21, page 212, in which the records of 160 patients sampled from over 5000 were examined for information on seven selected topics. As an example of an ambitious prospective audit one might sample 10% of hospital referrals—for example, table 12, page 208—and seek additional information from the referring doctor during the initiating consultation, the hospital consultant during the first outpatient visit, and the patient by post after discharge from the outpatient clinic.

The first step in sampling is to define the *population*—the entire set of items or measurements of interest.[1] To audit the treatment within a practice of a chronic primary disease such as asthma or diabetes, for example, one might define the population as all patients in the practice with the specified condition. For an acute illness such as childhood vomiting, however, a more appropriate population may be patients who consult the doctor about that illness within a given period. A *sample* is any subset of the population of interest that is used to draw conclusions about that population.

EXAMPLE 2—Fifty of the 725 hospital referrals in table 12, page 208, could be examined in detail by drawing one of the following samples (of which only the last is at all representative):
- the first 50 referrals in the year of interest
- half the patients referred by the trainee
- all the medical and geriatric referrals
- the first referral in each of 50 weeks in the year.

The process of drawing conclusions about a population from a sample is called *statistical inference*. The quality of the inference depends on both the sample size and how representative of the population the sample is.

Bias occurs when the sample is not representative of the population. It may occur at either or both of two stages: the definition of the *sampling frame*—a list of all the members of the population; and the choice of *sampling procedure*—the way in which items are selected from the sampling frame.

Sampling frames

The best sampling frame contains one and only one entry for each member of the population of interest. Most sampling frames, however, suffer from one or more of the following defects:
- Missing elements, which should be listed but are not
- Foreign elements, which should not be listed but are

- Duplicated elements—that is, many entries for one element
- Clustered elements—that is, one entry for many elements.

EXAMPLE 3—To sample from all episodes of illness in the practice the appointments book might be used as a sampling frame. This method would include all the defects above:
- Illnesses seen only by the practice nurse
- Patients who made appointments but did not attend
- Episodes of illness with two or more consultations
- Separate consultations for two or more family members within the same appointment.

EXAMPLE 4—To sample from all patients referred to hospital during 1989 copies of referral letters could be used as a sampling frame. There would probably be missing elements (for example, emergency admissions), foreign elements (for example, temporary residents), and duplicated elements (for example, patients referred more than once during the year), but there would probably be no clustered elements unless one letter was used to refer two or more patients.

As far as possible such errors should be corrected or allowed for; otherwise the sampling frame will not be representative of the population.

Sampling procedure

The aim is to make the sample representative of the sampling frame. *Judgment samples* are personally selected, often using a quota system. But they are usually unrepresentative, and statistical inferences are rarely safe. Therefore some form of *random sampling* will almost always be necessary; every item should have a chance of being selected.

In a *simple random sample* every possible sample, and therefore every item, has an equal chance of being selected. This can be done using a random number table (for example, that on page 9 of Bland[2]). The items in the sampling frame are numbered and those whose numbers occur in a chosen section of the random number table are taken as the sample. (It is not necessary to choose a random part of the table for each sampled item as consecutive digits are not related.)

EXAMPLE 5—To choose 20 out of 880 consultations for a given "tracer condition" (defined on pages 42–3) take 20 sets of three consecutive random digits, ignoring sets larger than 880 and sets that have already been drawn. As random numbers are equally likely to take any value the items in the sampling frame may be ordered in any convenient way—for example, alphabetical or chronological.

A *systematic sample* is quicker to obtain than a simple random sample; for instance, in example 5 one could choose one of the first 44 consultations at random and thereafter every 44th. This would also give 20 relevant consultations, but use only one random number. However, there is a risk of bias if, say, there are about 22 relevant consultations a week and Monday consultations differ from Friday consultations. Every sample item is equally likely to be chosen as each belongs to precisely one of the 44 possible samples.

Sample size

An unbiased sample chosen by a good sampling procedure from a good sampling frame will give estimates that are without a systematic tendency to be too large or too small. An individual estimate from a single sample, however, may diverge substantially from the *parameter* to be estimated (the true underlying value), especially if the sample is too small. Too small a sample will fail to label as *significantly* below the predetermined standard a performance that falls so far below that standard as to be *clinically* important. Too large a sample, as well as wasting effort, will label as significantly below standard a performance that is nevertheless close enough for the difference to be of no clinical importance.

EXAMPLE 6—Suppose that the desired standard for the vaccination rate among 2 year olds in the practice is 90%, that an actual rate as low as 80% is considered clinically important, and that you would like to detect such a departure from the standard on at least 95% of the occasions on which it occurs. Then statistical calculations along the lines described by Moser and Kalton[1] can be used to calculate the sample size needed: in this example it is about 133 children.

Note that this example could be interpreted as a criticism of a key element of the new contract, which takes no account of practice size when awarding target payments. A rate of only 85% in a small practice could be a random fluctuation from a "satisfactory" performance and a rate of 90% could be a random fluctuation from an "unsatisfactory" performance. Even worse, the clinically insignificant difference between 89% and 90% may be most significant financially.

Validity and reliability

As well as avoiding bias in the sample it is important to ensure that one is measuring what one wants to measure. It is desirable to check on this both in planning the audit and on a subsample of the patients whose care is being audited.

EXAMPLE 7—Blood pressure measurements vary according to the attitude of the patient (standing, sitting, or lying), the interval since exercise, and the identity of the measurer (doctor, nurse, or patient).[3] The diagnosis of asthma varies substantially between general practitioners.[4] When auditing the care of hypertension and asthma, two chronic conditions, both practices and standard setters should therefore use well defined diagnostic criteria.

Reliability measures internal consistency: if the measurement is repeated under the same conditions how much will it vary?

EXAMPLE 8—In example 7 repeated measurements by the same measurer on the same patient in the same attitude will provide a measure of reliability.

Validity measures consistency with the "gold standard." Is the measurement correct? If not how well does it correlate with the gold standard?

EXAMPLE 9—Even if the gold standard for blood pressure is based on measurement when the patient is lying down, measurement when the patient is standing can be used for audit if its bias is more or less consistent—for example, 10–20% above the lying measurement—but not if it is sometimes 20% below and sometimes 20% above.

Checking reliability

This is an important component of audit—often more important than checking validity. The methods available include the following.

(*a*) Repeated measurement—for example, of blood pressure. This is not always possible, however. For instance, the reliability of a questionnaire on patients' knowledge of asthma cannot usefully be tested by sending second copies of the questionnaire to the same patients, as this is likely merely to test the patients' memories of their previous answers.

(*b*) Measurement by another partner or member of the primary care team—for example, to confirm the accuracy with which an outcome like hearing loss has been measured.

173

(c) Measurement by another method, such as a postal questionnaire to the patient or a self administered blood sugar reading.
Of these methods the first is likely to show the smallest variation.
But it may not be superior to the other methods if it causes too
much reliance to be placed on a measurement whose value is highly
dependent on who is doing the measuring. If Dr A always
measures blood pressure when the patient is standing, and Dr B
measures it when the patient is lying down, knowledge of the
measurement alone is not an adequate guide to whether a patient
should be classified as hypertensive.

Checking validity

Although the gold standard is sometimes available in general
practice, checking validity will more often entail direct comparison
with hospital or laboratory data.

Analysing the data

The purpose of analysing the data from a practice audit is to
compare results from that practice with a fixed standard so as to
answer the question: "Is the practice meeting the standard for this
activity?" There may also be a subsidiary question: "By how much
do we fall short of the standard?"

If only a sample of the relevant patients is used *statistical
analysis* is needed to draw inferences about the population from the
sample. Even if all relevant patients are used statistical analysis will
still be appropriate if these patients represent a sample from the
population of all patients who could have suffered from the
condition that is the subject of the audit. Inferences may be of
three types, depending on the sample data.
(1) There is significant evidence that practice performance is
below the standard.
(2) There is significant evidence that practice performance is
above the standard.
(3) There is insufficient evidence that practice performance differs
from the standard.

The choice between (1), (2), and (3), or more realistically
between (1) and (3), needs a *hypothesis test*.[2] If an answer to the
subsidiary question is also needed a *confidence interval*[5] is appropriate.

174

EXAMPLE 10—Suppose the practice has decided to aim for a standard that requires that 70% of male patients between 30 and 45 should have had their blood pressures recorded within the past five years. Suppose further that in a sample of 100 such patients only 60 records show such a reading. Can we infer that the practice is not meeting the standard?

If the practice is meeting the standard precisely then on average a sample of 100 patients will include 70 "successes" (patients whose blood pressure has been recorded). We would not be at all surprised if there were 69 or 71 successes but we do expect the number of successes to be close to 70.

There are thus two possible explanations for the observed success rate of 60%:

(a) The practice is meeting the standard but an unlikely event has occurred: we have chosen a sample in which only 60 patients have their blood pressure recorded, rather than the 70 patients that might have been expected.

(b) The practice is not meeting the standard; fewer than 70% of all male patients in the practice have had their blood pressure recorded.

The usual statistical approach is to accept the first explanation unless the chance of the "unlikely event" is extremely small, typically less than 5%. If so the second explanation is preferred to the first and conclusion (1) applies: the proportion of male patients whose blood pressure has been recorded is *significantly* below 70%. If, however, the "unlikely event" is not so very unlikely, occurring in rather more than 5% of practices that are meeting this standard, conclusion (3) will apply: there is insufficient evidence to say that the practice is not meeting the standard; the proportion of male patients whose blood pressure had been recorded is not significantly below 70%.

Provided that the sample of 100 patients has been randomly chosen, we can use the mathematical theory of variation among repeated samples from the same population to calculate the chance of the "unlikely event" occurring. This is one of the strongest arguments for using random samples; in a judgment sample, even if the bias is not large, there is no way of calculating how unlikely an atypical sample is.

If a random sample of size n is taken from a population in which the proportion of successes is p then the average size of the *sample* proportion will also be p. Here $n = 100$ and $p = 0.7$ (70%). The larger the sample size, the closer to p the sample proportion is

175

likely to be. The variability of the sample proportion is measured by its *standard error*—a measure of the likely difference between sample and population proportions. The formula for this standard error is

$$\sqrt{[p(1-p)/n]}.$$

Thus for a sample of size 100, from a population with success rate of 0.7, the standard error of the sample proportion is

$$\sqrt{(0.7 \times 0.3/100)} = \sqrt{0.0021} = 0.046\ (4.6\%).$$

If the sample size is larger (say, 400) the average size of the sample proportion is still 0.7, but the standard error is smaller:

$$\sqrt{(0.7 \times 0.3/400)} = 0.023\ (2.3\%).$$

If the sample size is smaller (say, 40) the standard error is larger:

$$\sqrt{(0.7 \times 0.3/40)} = 0.072\ (7.2\%).$$

The actual sample of 100 patients has a sample proportion of 0.6 (60%), which is 0.1 (10%) below the agreed standard. To find out how likely such a difference between population and sample is we compare the observed difference of 0.1 with the standard error of 0.046. We note that the sample proportion is 2.17 standard errors smaller than the population proportion of 0.7 required to meet the standard.

Statistical tables (for example, that on page 121 of Bland[2]) show that a value of 2.17 or higher has a probability of only 0.015 (1.5%). The chance that a sample from a practice that is meeting the standard will have as few as 60 out of 100 successes is only 1.5%. This chance is much less than the usual criterion of 5%. Thus rather than believing that such an unlikely event has occurred we prefer to conclude that *the proportion of male patients whose blood pressure has been recorded is significantly below 70%*. There is evidence (at the 5% level) that the practice is not meeting the standard. (See conclusion (1) on page 174.)

If there were only 40 patients in the sample, with 24 successes, then the sample proportion would still be 0.6—that is, 0.1 below the standard. But the standard error would be 0.072, with the result that the sample proportion would be only 1.39 standard errors smaller than the agreed standard of 0.7.

The same statistical tables[2] show that a value of 1.39 or higher has a probability of 0.082 (8.2%). As this is larger than the usual criterion of 5% it should be concluded that the "unlikely event" is not sufficiently unlikely to reject explanation (*a*). A sample of this size might well estimate the success rate at 60% or below even if the practice were meeting the standard. So here we prefer explanation (*b*) and conclude that *the proportion of male patients whose blood pressure has been recorded is not significantly different from 70%.* There is not enough evidence (at the 5% level) to state that the practice is not meeting the standard.

Note the difference between the two cases: although both samples have the same proportion of successes, this is judged to be significantly below the standard only in the first case, since the larger the sample size the less the population and sample are likely to differ.

EXAMPLE 11—Example 6 suggested that a sample size of 133 was needed to compare a practice vaccination rate with an agreed standard of 90%. Provided that a sample of this size is achieved, calculations similar to those described in example 10 would establish that a sample vaccination rate of 85% or less was significantly below the desired standard of 90%. Sample rates lower than 85% are unlikely to occur when the practice as a whole is meeting the standard. A sample rate between 86% and 90% is not, however, considered sufficiently unlikely in a practice that is meeting the standard to justify the conclusion that the practice as a whole is not meeting the standard.

If the practice has an "unsatisfactory" rate of only 80% this will be detected unless the *sample* happens to have a vaccination rate above 85%—higher than the overall practice rate. The sample size of 133 has been chosen so that such a practice is detected as unsatisfactory on 95% of the occasions on which this occurs.

Confidence intervals for example 10—The best estimate for the true rate of blood pressure recording in the practice is 60/100 (60%). Many other true population percentages, however, could have given rise to the sample we have observed. If the sample is not biased the most likely such population percentages are close to 60% and the least likely are much larger or smaller than 60%.

A *confidence interval*[5] gives a range of population percentages that is likely (usually 95% or 99% likely) to include the true one.

The upper and lower limits of such an interval can be calculated from an approximate formula that uses the standard error introduced in example 10. If q is the proportion (percentage divided by 100) observed in a sample of n patients then it is

(a) 95% certain that the population proportion is between

$$q - 1.96\sqrt{[q(1-q)/n]} \quad \text{and} \quad q + 1.96\sqrt{[q(1-q)/n]}$$

(b) 99% certain that the population proportion is between

$$q - 2.58\sqrt{[q(1-q)/n]} \quad \text{and} \quad q + 2.58\sqrt{[q(1-q)/n]}.$$

Confidence levels other than 95% or 99% can be obtained by replacing the multipliers 1.96 or 2.58 by another from statistical tables.[2]
Here

$$q = 0.6 \quad \text{and} \quad \sqrt{[q(1-q)/n]} = 0.049.$$

Thus a 95% confidence interval for the true rate of blood pressure recording in the practice lies between $(0.6 - 1.96 \times 0.049)$ and $(0.6 + 1.96 \times 0.049)$—that is, between 0.504 and 0.696 (50.4% and 69.6%). A 99% confidence interval lies between 47.5% and 72.5%. Although the second interval is wider it is more likely to include the true rate.

Types of test

Example 10 gives a test of a single proportion from a "large" sample. Different tests arise from different types of data and sizes of sample. For other tests and the conditions under which they are valid one should consult a standard statistics textbook.[2] Conclusions usually take the form of a *confidence interval*[5] for a practice percentage, average, or other parameter of interest, and a statement about practice performance similar to (1), (2), or (3) on page 174, associated with the relevant significance level.

Note that statement (3) does *not* imply that the standard is being met, merely that the evidence is not strong enough to say that it is not being met. If the confidence interval is extremely wide the sample size is probably too small. The best remedy is to take a larger sample, preferably of the size suggested by calculations like those reported in example 6.

Presenting the audit

Target audience

You will gain more from your audit if results are summarised in tables or graphs and conclusions clearly stated. In addition, you will often wish to present your findings to colleagues within the practice—for example, when suggesting changes. You may also wish to send a report to the local medical audit advisory committee.

Structure of report

The traditional structure for medical publications provides a useful basis for an audit report:
(1) Summary—a few hundred words to tell the reader
    (*a*) which standard you adopted
    (*b*) how your performance compared with it
    (*c*) how you now propose to bring your performance closer to your standard (revised if necessary).
(2) Introduction, with particular reference to
    (*a*) which topic you chose and why
    (*b*) which standard you adopted and why.
(3) Method, covering at least five basic components:
    (*a*) basic design (what you did in general terms)
    (*b*) sampling (how?)
    (*c*) data collection (how?)
    (*d*) data validation (how you checked your data and with what result)
    (*e*) analysis (how you compared your performance with the standard.
(4) Results, using tables or graphs where appropriate.
(5) Discussion, critically appraising both your audit method and your performance.
(6) Conclusions and recommendations, in particular
    (*a*) whether your standard should now be revised
    (*b*) how you propose to bring your performance closer to it.

The case for tables

A table is an effective way to summarise a set of figures. As an example compare the following paragraph with table 1 (both derived from table 2, page 203), by combining counties).

179

TABLE 1

	Doctor			
Age group	DAH	PJD	ADG	MAP
64 or less	1412	1191	793	1260
65–74	239	141	45	193
75 or more	203	90	51	152

On 1 January 1989 Dr DAH had 1412 patients under 65, 239 aged between 65 and 74, and 203 older patients; Dr PJD had 1191 patients under 65, 141 aged between 65 and 74, and 90 aged 75 or older; Dr ADG had 793 patients under 65, 45 between 65 and 74, and 51 aged over 75; and Dr MAP had 1260 patients aged 64 or less, 193 aged between 65 and 74, and 151 aged 75 or older.

Even this table can be improved as the following guidelines for tables suggest.

How to present tables

(1) Give the table a title that is helpful and clear but as concise as possible; label rows and columns even more concisely.

(2) It is usually best to put figures to be compared in a single column rather than in a single row.

(3) Where possible use a systematic ordering—for example, by size—so that patterns are easier to spot.

(4) Row or column totals or averages will often help interpretation.

(5) Row or column percentages will often help comparison, but do make the table more cumbersome.

(6) All percentages need either a numerator or a denominator; if "75% of patients were cured" there may only have been four patients.

(7) In presentation (but *not* in your original working documents) round figures to two (or exceptionally three) *effective* digits; later digits are almost always irrelevant and confuse the reader.

(8) Include the name and result of any statistical tests you use, preferably without using asterisks, $p < 0.05$, or other statistical jargon.

EXAMPLE 12—Applying criteria (1) to (4) to table 1 would give table 2. Applying criteria (5) to (8) to table 2 would give table 3.

TABLE 2—Patient numbers by doctor and age group

	Age group			
Doctor	64 or less	65–74	75 or more	Total
DAH	1412	239	203	1854
MAP	1260	193	152	1605
PJD	1191	141	90	1422
ADG	793	45	51	889
Total	4656	618	496	5770

Source: Family practitioner committee figures for 1 January 1989.

TABLE 3—Patient numbers by doctor and age group

	Age group						
	64 or less		65–74		75 or more		
Doctor	No	%	No	%	No	%	Total
DAH	1400	76	240	13	200	11	1900
MAP	1300	79	190	12	150	9	1600
PJD	1200	84	140	10	90	6	1400
ADG	800	89	45	5	50	6	890
Total	4700	81	620	11	500	9	5800

Differences between doctors are significant at the 0.1% level (chi-squared = 84 with 6 degrees of freedom).
Source: Family practitioner committee figures for 1 January 1989.

Note that the percentages were calculated from the original figures of table 2, not the rounded figures of table 3. Also the percentages in the bottom row of table 3 add up to 101% because they have been rounded to the nearest whole number; the last two were just over 10.5% and just over 8.5%. Similarly the rounded figures within table 3 do not add up exactly to the row and column totals.

Including percentages in table 3 has highlighted the differences between the age distributions of patients registered with the four doctors. The result of the significance test has confirmed the visual impression that the four distributions differ considerably.

The case for and against graphs

As an alternative to table 3 the data could be presented graphically. Figures 1 and 2 show two possible graphs. Figure 1 is a bar chart of

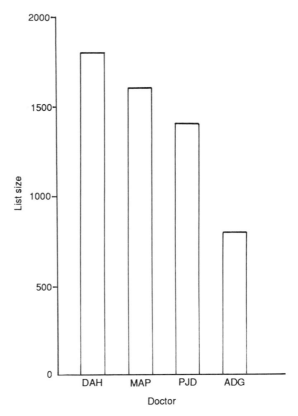

FIGURE 1—List sizes for the four doctors in the practice. (*Source*:Family practitioner committee figures for 1 January 1989.)

the list sizes for each doctor and figure 2 is a bar chart with three age-specific bars for each doctor and the height of each bar representing percentage.

Such graphs are good at highlighting one or two features but cannot include as much detail as a table without becoming confusing; for instance, figure 2 (already complex) does not include the relative sizes of the four doctors' lists.

Graphs are particularly good at illustrating trends. Figure 3 gives results from table 14, page 209, in graphical form. Both relative costs and differences in trends between the costs of different items are clearly seen.

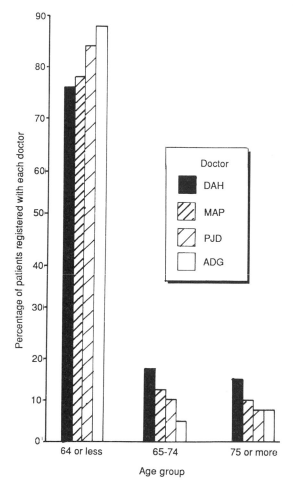

FIGURE 2—Age distribution of patients of the four doctors. (*Source*: Family practitioner committee figures for 1 January 1989.)

Conclusion

Our co-authors have argued that medical audit has great potential to improve primary medical care in the United Kingdom. We believe that both its validity and its effectiveness can be enhanced by careful attention to the basic statistical principles of sampling, data validation, analysis, and presentation.

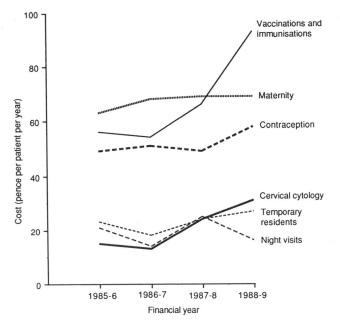

FIGURE 3—Item of service claims: cost per patient per year.

1 Moser CA, Kalton G. *Survey methods in social investigations.* 2nd ed. Aldershot: Gower, 1971.
2 Bland M. *An introduction to medical statistics.* Oxford: Oxford University Press, 1987.
3 Jamieson MJ, Webster J, Phillips S, et al. Measurement of blood pressure: Sitting or supine? Once or twice? *J Hypertension* 1990; **8**:635–40.
4 Speight ANP, Lee DA, Hay EN. Underdiagnosis and undertreatment of asthma in childhood. *Br Med J* 1983;286:1256–8.
5 Gardner MJ, Altman DG. *Statistics with confidence.* London: British Medical Journal, 1989.

Small group work

MAIRI SCOTT, MARSHALL MARINKER

Introduction

What is a small group? Definitions abound and contradict one another but for the purposes of this chapter we shall define it as a group of between five and 15 people who meet to carry out some agreed enterprise. Eight is often considered the optimum number. These figures are not as arbitrary as might be thought. If the group becomes too small—four or fewer—the possibility of different interactions limits creativity, encourages the taking of fixed roles, and creates too cramped a space for strong feelings to be safely aired or for strong personalities to be moderated by group behaviour. Too large a number and the cohesion of the group begins to break up; for example, it becomes impossible for all the members of a large group to be aware of the behaviour of all the others. In particular, whoever leads a small group must be aware of the behaviour of all of its members. If he or she cannot remain in visual contact with all the members, is unable to notice the eagerness of one, the melancholy of another, the puzzlement or anger or frustration that any group member may exhibit at any time, it will be impossible to address the given task or to deal with the problems within the group that this task may engender.

In the one to one relationship between mother and child, between husband and wife, between master and apprentice there can be a passion, a connectedness, an acuteness of feeling that cannot be replicated with the same intensity beyond the private confines of a two person "group." Small groups can certainly generate their own emotional storms: social psychologists of a variety of schools have suggested how and why these come about and these issues will be raised later in this chapter. But there is also something about the configuration of a small group that can exercise a profoundly civilising influence on the relationships of its members.

Thinking and feeling

As members of small groups what is required of each of us is that we find a place, a voice, a part to play in a shared enterprise. To achieve this we have to explore the minds, the thinking, and the feeling of a number of other people. If the enterprise of the group is to succeed we have to understand the strengths of others so that we can make these part of our own strength. We have to explore weaknesses but only so that we can compensate for them. None of this is possible unless each individual begins to reflect on the self. What do I know and how do I know it? What are my capacities and what are their limits? What are the values that drive me, the fears that haunt me? Who am I?

For the most part we are born into small groups. As children we are given the opportunity to play in small groups and, although most of our schools force us into the larger crowd of the classroom, schoolchildren play in small groups and team sports echo this primal expression of the hunter band.

In general practice, as in so many other walks of life, small groups abound: partnerships; primary health care teams; the families of patients; professional committees; and of course small group learning in vocational training and continuing medical education. Each of these groups differs from every other in terms of its structure, its distribution of authority, its explicit intentions, and its implicit rules of engagement. And yet each bears a strong family resemblance to all the others.

Small group work depends above all on a sensitivity to personal boundaries. It demands the ability to fit into the organisation and to make appropriate space for others. Each member of the group needs the tolerance of others if he or she is to venture his or her own ideas, ideals, or feelings. Members of the group can best achieve this tolerance by working hard to create tolerance for the ideas, ideals, and feelings of the others.

It should not surprise us that groups so often fail—for example, general practice partnerships can become frozen in glacial antagonisms. Past quarrels and unresolved misunderstandings from years—sometimes from decades—past survive frozen fresh but dead in ice packed hatred. Marriages and families can be like this; so can our medicopolitical committees. Other groups in trouble suggest a different metaphor. Groups can seem stuck in the groove of a cracked record. Some of the members seem mesmerised by the sound of the voices of the others; some are no longer listening; some find good reason to forget the next meeting; too late, someone suggests trying a new record or switching off the machine.

Tasks

In an essay on medical audit one of us (Marinker 1986)[1] stated that the following functions would be required from those taking part in the process:

- Determining what aspects of current work are to be observed and measured
- Measuring present performance and trends
- Determining priorities in terms of what is to be changed
- Negotiating these priorities with colleagues, including colleagues in other health care professions, and with client groups
- Developing specific standards of care. This will include an evaluation of the results of good empirical research and the logic of argument where objective evidence for choices is scant
- Negotiating these standards with colleagues
- Monitoring and controlling these standards
- Deciding the frequency of reviews
- Deciding the range, category, and number of standards to be subjected to medical audit
- Deciding about intraprofessional, interprofessional, and public accountability
- Exploring the value system that underpins these choices. These values will touch on public and private morality, the personal and public cost of health care, specific cost effectiveness, quality of life, and so on
- Resolving the many conflicts that arise from the expected variety of values expressed and beliefs held.

Many of these functions, particularly those involving cooperative tasks such as negotiating and resolving conflicts, are best tackled in small groups. In general practice we rarely think of the partnership, or even the primary health care team, as a small group. The term "small group" is more usually reserved for more formal occasions, usually concerned with some educational enterprise. Medical audit, however, is at one and the same time an indispensable management tool for modern general practice, a research into the functioning of the practice, and an intensive learning experience for all who become involved. If medical audit is to become an integral part of clinical practice and practice management, indeed if it is to function both as the intellectual and organisational framework of the practice, those who take part in it will need from time to time to constitute themselves into formal small groups. There is no other way in which the partnership, or the partners together with the practice manager and other key personnel, can discuss their aims for the practice, the priorities which they wish to choose, the aspects of the practice which are to be observed, and so on. Only by developing the skills of small group membership and leadership can the members of the practice become at once efficient, effective, open, and creative.

Work and avoidance

When a group works successfully at its task, when it shares and addresses its avowed aims, there will be few problems about behaviour or group processes. But sometimes, and not infrequently, the dynamics of the group far from helping actually impede good work. What is going on when things go wrong? What should the leader do?

When things go wrong inside a group it is most comfortable to look first for reasons outside. External ascription of such things as fault, blame, or incompetence does more than defend the amour propre of members of the group: it allows them to avoid looking at relationships and it may give them an important sense of cohesiveness, which like all seductions may prove misleading.

One influential model of small group dynamics comes from psychoanalysis. Bion[2] talks about *the work group* and *the basic assumption group*. The characteristics of both these groups, he maintains, are usually present at the same time.

The work group is concerned with the avowed aims. Small group learning in psychoanalysis and related psychologies is concerned with what in general practice we would call case discussion. A work group simply discusses the case and its implications. In particular the work group does not change the subject. When the group begins to change the subject Bion describes it as a basic assumption group. The basic assumption group is concerned with a different belief about what it is that the group has come together to do.

Bion identifies three sorts of behaviour in basic assumption groups. The first is *dependency*. Here the group assumes that the leader will be powerful and omniscient. The leader is seen to be there to solve problems. Balint and others suggest that there is an analogy here with the naive relationship between the general practitioner and the consultant—although this sounds rather old fashioned now. The second is described as *flight–fight*. Here the basic assumption is that the group has enemies without and that the role of the leader is to identify external danger and help the group run away from it. Alternatively he may locate the enemy and engage the group in a fight. Group cohesiveness is the aim and paranoia the method. Thirdly, Bion describes *pairing*. The manifestation of this is the development of a dialogue or a series of dialogues within the group. If the leader has been identified the dialogue may occur with the leader. Here the basic assumption of the group is that out of such dialogues (which psychoanalysts of course relate to some sort of sexual union) something good and hoped for and fruitful will be born.

It is worth while remembering that the original model stemmed from the attitudes of psychoanalysis and concerned the function of psychoanalytical therapy groups. This must limit the relevance of the model to our current needs. Pierre Turquet and Robert Gosling,[3] writing about Balint seminars, used the model to explain why groups of hard working and sophisticated doctors who had come together to achieve a specific and important task chose to spend a considerable amount of time and effort on a quite different task: the survival and integrity of the group itself.

Small groups and committees

There is a superficial resemblance between small groups and committees; for example, the size of many committees may be similar to the size that we might expect of a small group. Moreover, it is sometimes easier to understand the behaviour of committees not in terms of their agendas, the power of argument, or the elaborate protocols of committee decision taking but more persuasively in terms of basic assumption groups: dependency, flight–fight, pairing, and so on. Despite these superficial resemblances committees and small groups are quite different kinds of human organisation.

For the most part the members of a committee, however committed to their agenda, come to that agenda with outside affiliations. These affiliations may be stronger and more important than the internal affiliation—that is, the affiliation to the other members of the group and to the agenda. An obvious example would be a liaison committee between two professional organisations. Most committees, however, exhibit this conflict between external and internal affiliation. Members of a committee are often elected to represent a variety of associated constituencies. Each of them may legitimately expect to have his or her own geographical, political, or pressure group interests advanced. This is the essence of committee work. But it is quite different from the essence of small group work.

The way in which a task is presented also differs markedly between committee and small group. The intentions of the small group meeting are most usually stated in broad terms. In medical audit the task might be case discussion or constructing a protocol for the management of patients with psoriasis or deciding what the practice would regard as a reasonable policy on accessibility. The task of the small group may be best seen as the intended destination of a journey. The culture of the group will determine how the journey is to be undertaken: what sort of route will be chosen, what sort of equipment required, who will act as scout, who will be in charge of provisions, who will monitor progress. Small group work does not begin with a route map, with an inventory of the necessary equipment and provisions, still less with marching orders. The creativity of the small group, its ability to solve problems in an unusual way, and, most precious of all, its ability pleasantly to surprise itself are based on the assumption that the journey and how it is to be accomplished can be known only when the group starts to work.

Committees have a different kind of task and a quite different approach. The intentions of a committee must be laid out in fine detail in a written agenda. Those of us who have attended committees where this preliminary work has been neglected know only too well that progress soon becomes impossible. Ideally, committee work is supported by detailed documentation and the members of the committee come armed with argument and counter argument. Only in this way can members of the committee be true to their outward affiliations.

It is possible for the same people to come together at one time as a committee and at another time as a small group. Indeed this may be vital for the proper management and development of general practice. Practice meetings concerned with administration and managerial decisions will certainly need the discipline of a committee meeting. A practice meeting concerned with medical audit may well take as its starting point such a vital question as "What is the practice here to do?" The meeting can succeed in tackling such a question only if it functions not as a committee but as a small group.

Nothing illustrates more clearly the difference between committee work and small group work as the difference between committee chairman and group leader. The chairman begins the meeting not only having achieved considerable control over the agenda but with a formulated view about the decisions that have to be taken. In a sense the chairman begins the meeting with a comprehensive, although still concealed, intention about the minutes that are to be written. The task of the committee members is to challenge these implicit minutes and when possible to change them in the direction that each committee member desires. The major tactic of all members of the committee, including its chairman, is advocacy. However urbane the meeting, however restrained the decorum, there is an inherently adversarial relationship between a committee and its chairman. Far from being a criticism of committees this description reveals its important strengths.

Leaders

The relationship between a group leader and the group contrasts sharply with that between the chairman and the committee. Far from being adversarial the relationship is intended to be cooperative. The tactic of the leader is to ensure that the group works on its agreed task and that it is made aware when there is deviation from that task. He or she should point out why and how the group has begun to escape from what it set out to do and so enable it to return to its purpose. As leader he or she is a resource person for small group work. He or she is not necessarily a resource person for the task being undertaken. That role may fall to another member of the group or indeed to all the members. It is important to bear in mind this distinction between the role of leader and the role of resource. The member of the practice who is most knowledgeable about medical audit may not necessarily be the person best equipped to lead the group.

The question of who is to lead the group is a delicate one. There are perhaps four issues that need to be considered when making a choice.

The first issue concerns *status*. Small group leadership may be charismatic, imposed, democratic, or sapiential. Where leadership is charismatic the leader may have a strong and attractive personality—the ability to disarm and persuade. The strengths and weaknesses of such a basis for leadership are self evident. Such leadership can be powerful, but its intentions can be idiosyncratic and self indulgent.

Leadership can be imposed: the leader may be appointed, for example, by a government or a university department. Again there are strengths and weaknesses. In such a situation the leader has clear accountability to the organisation under whose aegis the group is meeting, but because the leadership is imposed it exhibits a rigid fragility.

The leadership may be democratic: the members of the group themselves may choose their leader. There is strength here in the sense of ownership that the group has of its leader—the sense of participation and negotiation. The weakness is that such leadership, if it is perceived to confront or to challenge the group, can be terminated at the will of the group; so the leader is captive to the group's approval.

Leadership can be sapiential: the leader is recognised because he or she has knowledge or skills that the group wishes to acquire. Again the strength is one of ownership, participation, and negotiation. The weakness is that the group members may settle for a teacher–pupil relationship, a dependency from which too much is hoped for, and from which too much disappointment may ensue.

The status of the leader, of course, is never so categorically defined as these four archetypes suggest. But the archetypes need constantly to be borne in mind when problems with the leader arise.

The second issue concerns the *performance* of the leader. There are various styles of leadership, and these can profoundly affect both the feelings in the group and the group's ability to solve problems. The leader may exhibit an authoritarian, a sensitive, a forceful, or a laissez faire style. There is no such thing as the most effective style. Each group must discover what kind of leadership suits it best. This is quite different from suggesting that each group must discover what kind of leadership is least confronting or most comfortable. Once the leader begins to collude with the group, work is avoided and tensions will rise.

The third issue concerns the *orientation* of the leader. The leader may reveal an orientation towards an individual member of the group or to some particular members; there may be an orientation to the group as a whole and its interactions or there may be an orientation first and foremost to the task that the group has agreed to undertake.

The fourth issue certainly reflects on the personality of the group leader; but it also reflects on the relationship between the leader and the group. What is the *culture* of the group? What are the values, perhaps never stated explicitly nor examined critically, that the group expresses?

Groups sometimes exhibit a strong work ethic with the members showing impatience or even intolerance to those who wish to deflect attention from the task in hand. Other groups value relationships far more than the tasks. If a member is in difficulty all attention to the task must stop while a rescue mission is organised, executed, and brought to a successful conclusion.

These descriptions and differences are of course exaggerations, but they may provide some references for the exploration of your own small group work.

Conclusion

This chapter is intended to give only a partial description of small group work and to relate this to the tasks of medical audit. Much of the book is concerned with the ideas of medical audit, the frames of reference that may be used, the intellectual disciplines that have to be exercised. But the reader will already have detected behind these explorations of theory the passionate feelings and the strained relationships that are likely to be encountered. Even at the outset, when the partnership begins to think about its priorities, about what is to be audited, about what constitutes good general practice, the deeply held values of each individual must be challenged. What begins as a search for good standards of care for patients may quickly be transformed into a battle of wills between powerful antagonists.

Most groups concerned with medical audit will not be strangers to one another. This is both good and bad news. The good news is that little time needs to be spent on the preliminaries of small group induction: negotiating relationships, presenting abbreviated and acceptable biographies, and marking out territory. The bad news is that all the past feelings of the members about one another, old scores unsettled, hopes disappointed, opposing moral judgments, and so on may come to the surface with renewed force. Not only will there be interpersonal problems of this nature but also problems between members of allied professions. All the vexing questions about gender, status, values, and accountability that characterise the experience of the so called primary health care team will be sharpened by the attempt to carry out medical audit.

If the group is to be successful in medical audit, or for that matter in any other part of the practice's endeavours, it will be helpful to understand what is going on beneath the surface of the discussion. In all this the task of the group leader is remarkably simple and its execution remarkably complex. The task is constantly to remind the members of the group that they are meeting to enhance the quality of the care of patients. What is complex is the means of achieving this without serious damage to the self image and dignity of every member of the group.

There is a limit to what can be learnt about small group work from written theory. As with learning to play a musical instrument or a good game of tennis one learns most by reflection in action. A good group leader can facilitate this reflection but all the members of the group have a part to play. Finally, it is worth remembering that most general practitioners have considerable interpersonal skills, which they deploy in their consultations. For some mysterious reason these skills desert them at meetings with partners or with other members of the primary health care team. Perhaps what we betray in this strange split between our work with patients and our work with colleagues is a naive belief that, while our patients are vulnerable and require understanding, we and our colleagues are tough and strong and must be feared rather than helped. The reader may regard this as a simplistic exaggeration. But if the idea has a ring of truth then it may point the way to a much gentler, much more humane, and in the end for more effective form of small group work within practices. There is no other way to assure the future success of medical audit.

1 Marinker M. Performance review and professional values. In: Pendleton D, Schofield T, Marinker M, eds. *In pursuit of quality*. London: The Royal College of General Practitioners, 1986.
2 Bion WR. *Experiences in groups*. London: Tavistock, 1986.
3 Gosling R, Miller DH, Woodhouse D, Turquet PM. *The use of small groups in training*. London: Codicote Press, 1964.

Practice reports

MICHAEL PRINGLE

Introduction

Practice reports are burgeoning.[1][2] From the first recorded example in Ballymoney Health Centre in 1969 they have developed from a minority pursuit to a feature of many progressive practices today.

Practice reports evolve.[2][3] A practice may start with a short account of its history, its current staff, and a few statistics, often supplied by the family practitioner committee or the Prescription Pricing Authority. Such early reports are quickly produced; they help to provide motivation and reward for effort. The result may lead to both satisfaction at a milestone achieved and dissatisfaction at the many unanswered questions raised.

In the second year the report may contain prevention and screening rates, consultation rates, and referrals, all of which require data collection, often continuously over a year. Later come accounts of investigation rates, chronic disease audits, and the practice finances. This evolution mirrors the developing information systems and appreciation of the value of information within the practice.

Practice reports vary widely. There may be common elements, but each report will be a disparate product of varying circumstances. Since the motivation comes from within the practice and the report is designed primarily to respond to a practice's needs, the contents and presentation can be idiosyncratic. As a practice looks beyond its boundaries it may need to compare itself to other practices and to local and national norms. If it does this it will need to use common definitions for the items it wishes to compare. Although the range and depth of a practice report will be determined by the needs and skills of the practice, there will be an increasing recognition of the value of standardisation for certain aspects

If it fulfils no other role a practice report must be of value to the practice for measuring the quantity and quality of care[4]; determining the use of, and need for, resources; and setting targets to which the practice can aspire.[5] To do this it must be honest, and honesty creates vulnerability. Each practice must decide how far it is willing to disseminate its report and whether it requires two versions. To be of value, in addition to being honest a report must be accurate, which requires the contents to be both quantitative—with numbers, percentages, and averages—and qualitative—with descriptions of how the practice is seen by its members. Further, it needs to be of sufficient depth to allow a reasoned analysis of the practice's problems and the solutions to them.

As practice reports follow on over the years they can be used to monitor developments, to record performance against targets, and to identify trends. Just as the computer is becoming an essential tool for data processing so the annual report will become a prerequisite for data presentation and understanding and thus an integral part of the management of a modern practice.

What is a practice report?

Any document that a practice produces which describes the working of the practice can be described as a practice report. Practice reports have, however, acquired some characteristics. They are usually produced annually; express a consensus view of the practice team; and are, at the least, available to every member of the team. Their contents may include a description of the practice philosophy, an analysis of the practice workload, an audit of clinical standards, and the setting of targets for the future.

A major confusion has been created by the use of the term annual report by the Department of Health in the new contract for general practitioners.[6] Although annual reports can be seen as one specialised form of practice report with an overlap in their contents, they are clearly philosophically different documents.

Annual reports to the family practitioner committee

Annual reports are now a contractual requirement. Therefore the need for them is not initiated by the practice and the practice may comply without realising that the information involved relates to any of its problems. This means that the first prerequisite of the educational audit process, an acknowledgement of a potential problem, is not present. The motivation within a practice for producing the report is contractual compliance, not honest self evaluation.

Contractual annual reports are intended to act as tools for minimum standard monitoring and as a weapon in the cost containment war, which is characterised by government sources as "value for money." Practitioners may unfortunately become wary of presenting information in a straightforward way, not only in annual reports but in any practice reports because they fear that the information may be used for punitive purposes either against themselves or other practitioners.

The family practitioner committee will require annual reports to contain details of staff and their training; practice premises and plans for their upgrading; the external commitments of the partners; and prescribing policy. The most onerous part, however, will be the reporting of referrals, including self referrals, both of inpatients and outpatients. This is to include pathology and x ray investigation requests.[7]

Practice reports

In the rest of this chapter we shall consider practice reports that are compiled voluntarily as an educational, clinical, and management audit. They are intended to throw light on the performance of the practice, both subjectively and objectively, so that the practice may evaluate itself in a spirit of self criticism. Such honesty inevitably creates vulnerability, and practices will only be prepared to tolerate such vulnerability if the risks are minimised. If there are strong fears that data gathered for internal educational audit could be used for making punitive external judgments—for monitoring the contract, determining earnings, or instituting litigation—practices will have a powerful motive for not preparing practice reports.

The content and format of practice reports are flexible. Practices need to choose where to start and the pace of their progress, but three theoretical stages can be postulated.

- *Stage 1. Description*—The practice describes its structure (personnel, premises, patients), and its process (reports from the primary health care team).
- *Stage 2. Process audit*—As well as describing itself, the practice audits and publishes its workload—that is, consultations, visits, clinics—referral and investigation rates, prevention levels and prescribing.

- *Stage 3. Clinical audit*—At this level the practice also publishes audits of its clinical protocols for common chronic diseases and special groups of patients.

Although some of the information in the annual report may reappear in the practice report—for example, referral and investigation rates—it will be serving a different purpose in a different context. Here I shall concentrate on the nature of this purpose and attempt to define the context.

What function does a practice report perform?

Internal function

The prime functions of a practice report should be internal to the practice. If it is compiled with a selfconscious look over the shoulder at the possible reactions outside the practice then its value inside the practice may well be compromised.

The practice report is above all a tool in the management of change. It is means of addressing the key questions below.[34]

- Where have we come from?
- Where are we now?
- Where are we going?
- How do we intend to get there?

Knowing where the practice has been helps in interpreting the present and highlighting trends that may continue. Target setting has to be based on an understanding of the past and the present; and deciding how the targets are to be achieved is of course essential.

Some practices go through this process in a somewhat disorganised way without the imposed structure of an annual report. So they risk seeing areas of practice activity in a piecemeal fashion and often fail to share their ideas with employees. Worst of all, they risk missing a stage, basing their perception of problems on insufficient data, and applying inappropriate solutions.

In one practice a series of complaints was received from patients about the availability of appointments: the patients had to wait too long for the first available appointment. Once identified this problem was openly and honestly discussed at a practice meeting and, as a longer term solution, it was agreed to take on an extra partner. In the meantime the practice decided to offer three extra appointments for each doctor in each morning surgery. But to everyone's surprise this short term solution did not work. So one partner and the practice manager set about auditing the problem. They found that the source of the problem was that patients had difficulty in contacting the practice because there was only one line. This made patients frustrated and irritable. Morning appointments were the last to be booked and were often left vacant. Evening appointments were in considerable demand and it was the lack of these that was causing the problem. It therefore became clear that the first solution, although apparently reasonable, had not addressed the real problem, which was defined by a simple audit.

For many practices change is not something they bring about but something that happens to them. They are reactive in a proactive world and this passivity results in their being left increasingly behind. Starting a practice report is one way of changing the culture of a practice from being reactive to proactive.

A practice report has other internal functions. It can inform the staff and patients of the activities of the practice; and it can mark the practice's achievements—it can acknowledge effort and excellence. By increasing awareness and understanding of the practice's goals it can draw the partners, staff, and patients into an involvement that leads to high staff morale; thriving patient groups; a coherent working relationship between partners; and the achievement of targets.

External functions

In setting targets a practice has to make judgments based on the present. Only if it has access to normative data from other practices with which it can compare its performance can it make reasoned judgments. By publishing its report externally each practice will help others to set their norms.

By making practice reports common currency we shall be able to make our peer reviews meaningful. To judge a practice using statements made ex cathedra by a central body is a limited exercise, but to compare practices by using the norms of other similar practices gives peer review credibility. It is far better that central norms[8]—for example, as outlined in the Royal College of General Practitioners' guide to assessment for fellowship[9]—should be based on the real performances of real practices.[10]

The need for accountability to our patients[11] is another important motive for preparing practice reports. Although our peers may judge us by the profession's criteria, our patients should be able to judge us by their own criteria. An openness about our performance, whatever the shortcomings of that performance may be, is far better than a smug silence.

Sharing information about our performance with patients creates an awareness in the practice population of its needs. This was precisely the purpose of the Medical Officer of Health's annual report before 1972—an examination of the needs of a population and the extent to which they were met.[12] This public health function is within the grasp of general practices using information technology to generate high quality audits.

The last external function that practice reports can perform is to defend the profession. We are open to the charges that we are not evolving, that we do not set standards, that we are not self critical, that we do not perform, and that we do not communicate with our patients. Practice reports can answer these criticisms both in individual practices and, collectively, nationally. We have hidden our lights for too long; practice reports are one way of raising the torch.

The areas to be covered in a practice report

Two reports or one?

If a practice report is to stimulate higher standards and a more focused management of change then it must be honest. If such honesty would compromise the practice then the dissemination of the report must be restrained. This might be the case with details of partnership earnings, for example, but might also include any information that bears directly on compliance with the general practice contract. Every practice should therefore produce an unexpurgated core report. If it decides that this report should not be circulated widely it can either produce a second, limited, edition for wide distribution or restrict the single report to a limited readership.

These issues need to be decided before the report is written. If, as happens in my practice, only one version of the report is written and it is available to everyone within the practice, including the patients who read copies put in the waiting room, and outside bodies, including other practices and the family practitioner committee, the style must be suitable for the potential readership. If patients are to read it some terms need defining, and the text needs to be undemanding.

Contents

In constructing reports practices, of necessity, start with a few items and build up. The three stages have already been listed. The complexity of the first report and the speed with which it is produced will depend on both the will of the practice and the sophistication of its information systems. The possible contents (table 1) are those that a practice might aspire to, and could achieve, at the time.[3]

TABLE 1—The contents of a practice report

The past	History and development of the practice
The broad aims	The practice objective
	The system of care
The current structure	Staff (including names, job titles, qualifications and training)
	Premises
	Patient demography—age/sex, location, turnover
The year in question	A log of significant events
	Reports of members of primary health care team
	Report from patient participation group
	Meetings in the practice
	Courses attended (for example, continuing medical education courses)
	Research and publications
	Teaching and training
The process of care	Consultation rates
	Investigation rates
	Referral rates
	Items of service claims
	Prescribing data
	Causes of death
	Prevalence of chronic disease
Prevention	Immunisation rates
	Cervical cytology uptake rates
	Child care surveillance
	Screening
Clinical care	Protocols and their audits
	Medical records
Finances	Income, health service and private
	Expenses
	Equipment purchased
Planning ahead	Achievement of last year's targets
	Needs in the community
	Perceived deficiencies in the practice
	Targets in the short, medium, and long term

The examples quoted in the text and the tables are from the second practice report (covering July 1988 to June 1989 and published in December 1989) from my own practice in Collingham, Newark, Nottinghamshire. This report is far from perfect and is held up not as a model of perfection but as an example.

Although some items in table 1 are self explanatory, others need elaboration. The heading, "History and development of the practice" may only appear in early reports. It is valuable both as an examination of the background of the practice and for human interest, something that is often given only scant consideration.

Our first report contained an account by a retired partner of the major developments and innovations in his working life until he retired at the end of the 1970s. For the second report one of the present partners recounted his experience over the past 10 years. Staff and patients alike can relate to these accounts and can learn about, or be reminded of, the practice's origins and evolution.

The *practice's objectives* should be global definitions of the practice's aspirations.[5] These objectives should include the practice philosophy, availability, accessibility, remit for chronic disease and prevention, organisation, and a wider role outside the practice. The *system of care* (appendix A) should be a clear statement of the way in which patient care is delivered in the practice. It should be based largely on job descriptions.

Patient demography should conform to the rules for presenting data set out later in this chapter. It should include patient numbers (table 2), location, and turnover (tables 3 and 4).

TABLE 2—Patient numbers (July 1988–June 1989)

Doctor	Nottinghamshire				Lincolnshire			
	65	65–74	≥75	Total	65	65–74	≥75	Total
DAH	1019	159	158	1336	393	80	45	518
MAP	864	141	113	1118	396	52	39	487
PJD	871	122	76	1069	320	19	14	353
ADG	562	36	49	647	231	9	2	242
Total	3316	458	396	4170	1340	160	100	1600
	(3224)	(439)	(346)	(4009)	(1300)	(176)	(105)	(1581)
Total number of registered patients	5770 (5590)							

Figures for the previous year are in parentheses.
Source: Family practitioner committee figures for 1 January 1989 (mid-year).

203

TABLE 3—Patient turnover (July 1988–June 1989, July 1987–June 1988)

Practice population	Total		Nottinghamshire		Lincolnshire	
	1988–89	1987–88	1988–89	1987–88	1988–89	1987–88
New patients registered	427	616	299	*	128	*
New babies	43	50	28	*	15	*
Total	470	666	327	*	143	*
Patients who left the practice	380	419	263	247	117	172
Deaths	81	61	62	48	19	13
Total	461	480	325	295	136	185
Increase in practice population based on these figures	9 (186)†					

* No data available. † Figure for 1987–88 in parentheses.

TABLE 4—Turnover as percentage of practice population (July 1988–June 1989, July 1987–June 1988)

	1988–89	1987–88
Babies	0·74	0·88
All new patients	8·1	11·7
Deaths	1·4	1·02
Patients who left the practice (including patients who died)	8·0	8·4

A vital part of any practice report should be *reports from members of the primary health care team*—the doctors, receptionists, practice and district nurses, health visitors, the school nurse, the counsellor, and in our case the attached physiotherapist. These reports can be linked to the report from the patient participation group (see appendix B) to give a descriptive picture of the workings of the practice from both sides of the reception desk.

To calculate the number of contacts between doctors and patients in a year (the consultation rates) for inclusion in the report one needs to know the number of surgery consultations and visits (table 5) and the number of clinic appointments and medicals (tables 6–8). When the contacts with the primary health care team are known the total number of contacts per patient per year can be calculated (tables 9 and 10).

TABLE 5—Doctor workload (July 1988–June 1989, July 1987–June 1988)

| Doctor | Number of consultations | | On call | | | | | Visits | | | | | |
| | | | Number of surgeries | 1st | 2nd | Total | | Routine | | Urgent | | Total | |
	1988–89	1987–88	1988–89			1988–89	1987–88	1988–89	1987–88	1988–89	1987–88	1988–89	1987–88
DAH	3 818	3 664	322	100·5	23·5	124	114	290	252	332	302	622	554
MAP	2 406	2 474	202	58·5	20	78·5	97·5	234	225	255	217	489	442
PJD	3 617	3 826	310	91	26·5	117·5	108·5	289	369	335	287	624	656
ADG	1 562	1 494	134	37	8	45	46	191	112	147	172	338	284
Trainee	2 884	2 859	277	78	1	79	80	59	123	279	258	338	381
Urgent cases*	1 436	1 494											
Total	15 723	15 811	1 245 (1 233)†	365 (356)†	79 (80)†	444	436	1 063	981	1 348	1 236	2 411	2 217

* Urgent cases are seen at the end of surgery by whichever doctor finishes first. The workload involved is therefore not allocated to individual doctors.
† Figures in parentheses are totals for 1987–88. In these cases no data were recorded for individual doctors.

TABLE 6—Medical examinations

	Number	
	1988–89	1987–88
July to September	13	13
October to December	10	4
January to March	20	10
April to June	15	22
Total	58	49

TABLE 7—Antenatal clinics (July 1988–June 1989, July 1987–June 1988)

	First		Routine	
Doctor	1988–89	1987–88	1988–89	1987–88
DAH	11	15	99	119
MAP	6	11	79	112
PJD	14	13	77	149
ADG	19	11	127	130
Trainee	3	6	18	36

TABLE 8—Other clinics (July 1988–June 1989, July 1987–June 1988)

	Number	
	1988–89	1987–88
Baby clinic assessments	133	109
Well man clinics	53	97
Well woman clinics	143	108

TABLE 9—Workload in the primary health care team estimated on patient contacts (July 1988–June 1989, July 1987–June 1988)

	Total patients seen	
	1988–89	1987–88
District nurses	8454	7138
Health visitors	2902	2154
Midwife	446*	908*
Physiotherapy	1613	1888

* Clinic

TABLE 10—Total workloads and contact rates (July 1988–June 1989, July 1987–June 1988)

	1988–89	1987–88
Total patient contacts by doctors	19 032	18 888
Average number of contacts between doctor and patient	3·28	3·32
Total patient contacts by rest of primary health care team	13 415	12 088
Total contacts per patient	5·60	5·45

TABLE 11—Investigations (July 1988–June 1989)

Total number of specimens sent to laboratory was 3795. (In the previous year the number was 3664)

Types of investigations requested	Number
Full blood count and/or erythrocyte sedimentation rate	856
Electrolytes and urea	351
Urine culture	458
Swab for culture	191
Random blood sugar and/or HbAl	207
Liver function tests	183
Thyroid function tests	205
International normalised ratio	141
Pregnancy tests	77
B-12 and folate	18
Serum iron	19
Stool culture	85
Fasting lipids	138
Calcium, phosphates, alkaline phosphates	10
Histology	23
Drug level	44
Cervical smears	471
Other	318

Investigation rates (table 11) should be broken down by investigation type and, unlike in our report, should include x rays. *Referral rates* should be by speciality and location (table 12). Our report fails to include emergency admissions although it does offer an analysis (not shown) of where the patients were referred.

Items of service claim rates (tables 13 and 14), numbers of patients on the *prescribing system* (tables 15 and 16), and *causes of death* (table 17) are straightforward but the latter two require premeditated data collection.

TABLE 12—Hospital referrals (July 1988–June 1989)

	Doctor					
	DAH	MAP	PJD	ADG	Trainee	Total
Breast	4	3	2	4	7	20
Cardiac	6	2	3	1	–	12
Chest	3	2	3	3	3	14
Dermatology	16	16	14	10	14	70
Ear, nose, and throat	21	12	15	3	11	62
Geriatrics	3	2	3	1	–	9
Gynaecology	25	13	13	25	11	87
Medical (general)	8	3	14	4	12	41
Neurology	–	1	4	–	–	5
Obstetrics	10	6	10	18	4	48
Ophthalmics	24	8	23	11	7	73
Orthopaedics	29	7	22	11	11	80
Paediatrics (medical and surgical)	3	3	2	5	–	13
Psychology and psychiatry	2	2	2	2	2	10
Rheumatology	4	1	5	1	1	12
Surgical	20	17	26	23	7	93
Urology	7	4	4	3	3	21
Others	17	11	12	8	7	55
Total	202	113	177	133	100	725
	(204)	(125)	(204)	(114)	(143)	(790)

Referral rate = 0·13 (0·14) per patient per year or 125 per 1000 (139 per 1000)
        patients per year
      = 0·03 (0·04) per contact between doctor and patient in a year

Figures for the previous year are in parentheses.

TABLE 13—Items of service claims per 1000 patients per quarter (in £)

	In practice	County average
Temporary resident, low rate	37·12	24·90
Temporary resident, high rate	32·52	18·46
Contraception	134·88	148·83
Coil claims	8·13	14·20
Maternity	190·29	277·82
Night visit fees	41·49	93·40
Cervical cytology	77·87	37·01
Vaccination and immunisation	237·10	167·63
Emergency treatment	21·50	3·37
Total	780·90	785·62

TABLE 14—Items of service claims per patient per year (in £)

	85–86	86–87	87–88	88–89	National average 1987–88
Temporary residents, all	0·23	0·18	0·24	0·27	0·21
Contraception, all	0·49	0·51	0·49	0·58	0·58
Maternity	0·63	0·68	0·69	0·69	0·94
Night visits	0·21	0·14	0·25	0·16	0·27
Cervical cytology	0·15	0·13	0·24	0·31	0·14
Vaccinations and immunisation	0·56	0·54	0·66	0·93	0·45
Total average per patient	2·27	2·18	2·57	2·94	2·59

TABLE 15—Repeat prescribing analysis: number of patients on the repeat prescribing system

Doctor	30 July 1989	30 June 1988
DAH	497	457
MAP	327	328
PJD	495	478
ADG	147	97
Total	1466	1360

TABLE 16—Repeat prescribing analysis: distribution of number of items prescribed

Number of items	30 July 1989			30 June 1988		
	Male	Female	Total	Male	Female	Total
1	212	271	483	195	246	441
2	162	216	378	152	213	365
3	91	124	215	90	119	209
4	59	86	145	53	91	144
5	36	64	100	33	47	80
6	19	31	50	20	26	46
7	25	15	40	14	18	32
8	7	20	27	8	12	20
9	6	8	14	7	8	15
10	6	8	14	3	5	8

TABLE 17—Causes of death (July 1988–June 1989, July 1987–June 1988)

	Number	
	1988–89	1987–88
Cancer	19	19
Cerebrovascular accident (stroke)	4	5
Chest infections	13	10
Chronic obstructive airways disease	3	–
Congestive cardiac (heart) failure	6	2
Coronary artery disease	16	12
Old age	8	3
Respiratory failure	1	–
Septicaemia	2	–
Unknown	1	3
Other	8	8
Total	81*	61

* Of these patients 57 died at home.

Prevention statistics include those for the target payments (tables 18,19, and 20) and other screening activities. Usually included are statistics for child care surveillance, blood pressure recording, tobacco and alcohol consumption observations (table 21), and cholesterol screening (table 22).

The distinction between process measures and *clinical audits* is that the latter involve a definition of clinical care against which the delivery of care is assessed. In our practice report we have published the *audits of protocols* in our care of well man and well woman clinics, cervical cytology (table 20) and rubella immunisation programmes, hypertension, asthma, diabetes, myxoedema, and hypercholesterolaemia (table 22 and box on page 213). We have also audited our *medical records* for the numbers with problem lists and those checked for the disease register (table 21).

The extent to which a practice wants to include *financial data* in its report will vary. If a separate practice report is being prepared for the partners only then can it include the full financial details, but since these are usually a duplicate of the accountant's report this may be unnecessary. It is, however, possible to highlight trends by using an arbitrary year as a base (equal to 100 as in retail price indices) and showing changes year by year (table 23). Data presented in this manner should be publishable to any readership.

TABLE 18—Immunisation status of preschool children in practice

	Number	Percentage
Audit of all children aged 2 in the practice on 1 June 1989 (n = 46)		
Completed pertussis	43	93
Completed DTP/DT/polio	46	100
Had MMR	39	87
Had MMR or measles	43	93
Audit of all children aged 3 in the practice on 1 June 1989 (n = 65)		
Completed pertussis	54	83
Completed DTP/DT/polio	65	100
Had MMR	57	89
Had MMR or measles	60	93
Audit of all children aged 5 in the practice on 1 June 1989 (n = 80)*		
Completed pertussis	64	82
Completed DTP/DT/polio	80	100
Had MMR	37	47
Had MMR or measles	75	96
Preschool booster	61	78

* The 5 year old cohort includes children who have just reached the age of 5. Many mothers bring their children at school entry; hence the figure of 78% for the preschool booster.

TABLE 19—Immunisation status of preschool children: local averages

	During first year of life		Before the age of 2
	Diphtheria, tetanus, and pertussis (%)	Pertussis (%)	Measles (%)
Newark and Sherwood District	82	75	83
All Central Nottinghamshire District Health Authority	77	71	75

TABLE 20—Cervical smear uptake and system for results at June 1989

Women who are registered with the practice aged 25–65 (n = 1525)	Number	Percentage
On the smear recall system	1404	92
Known to have had a hysterectomy	124	8
Those who have positively declined cytology	12	0·8
Those who are up to date on our system*	1049	69
Those who have had a smear in the past five years	1216	80

* Women up to the age of 45 who have had a smear test in the past three years and those over 45 who have had smear tests every five years.

TABLE 21—Audit on recording of occupation, smoking habits, blood pressure, etc

Ten random records (selected by the practice preventative care nurse) were examined for each sex in each 10 year age band, giving 160 records in all

Item recorded	16–25		26–35		36–45		46–55		56–65		66–75		76–85		86–95		Total
	M	F	M	F	M	F	M	F	M	F	M	F	M	F	M	F	
Occupation	1	5	6	3	6	2	3	0	4	6	3	0	0	0	0	0	39
Alcohol	4	7	5	7	4	4	5	5	7	6	4	6	5	3	6	3	81
Smoking	4	7	5	7	4	4	5	5	7	6	4	6	5	3	6	3	81
Weight	0	7	0	4	3	5	3	2	5	1	1	3	1	3	3	1	42
Blood pressure	3	8	2	7	9	7	6	9	9	6	7	8	9	8	9	9	116
Problem list	9	10	8	10	9	10	10	9	10	10	10	9	10	9	10	10	153
Checked for disease register	8	9	9	9	10	5	9	8	8	7	8	8	10	10	9	10	137

TABLE 22—Audit of hypercholesterolaemia (for January–June 1989)

Total number of patients screened	81
Number with family history of ischaemic heart disease or peripheral vascular disease	8
Number with a family history of hypercholesterolaemia	9
Number with xanthoma	0
Number with corneal arcus or xanthelasma	1
Number with hypertension	55
Number with other disease (for example, diabetes)	8

Number of records marked "HYP" = 77
Number of records marked "HDL" = 32 (for discussion of screening relatives)

Age (years) of patients tested (number of patients)	20 (5)	20–40 (10)	40–60 (47)	>60 (19)

Results:

cholesterol (mmol/l) (number of patients)	5·2 (3)	5·2–6·5 (28)	6·2–7·5 (28)	>7·5 (23)
triglyceride (mmol/l) (number of patients)	3·0 (77)	>3·0 (4)		

Number of patients tested who smoked	11
Number of these who had cholesterol levels >7·5 mmol l	4
Hypothyroidism	1
Number of patients with cholesterol >7·5 mmol/l investigated to exclude other causes	8

TABLE 23—Financial trends

	1984	1985	1986	1987	1988
Turnover	100	108	117	131	147
Total expenditure	100	98	118	128	140
Staff salaries and pensions	100	102	108	123	125
Office expenses and telephones	100	111	126	161	166
Total income	100	108	117	131	147
Profit	100	127	116	137	161

Based on indexation on 1984 as an arbitrarily chosen year.

Practice protocol for hypercholesterolaemia

Screening policy

We shall screen all those patients who are
- aged less than 60 with hypertension, ischaemic heart disease, diabetes, or myxoedema
- first degree relatives of patient with ischaemic heart disease or hypercholesterolaemia
- identified by doctor as having xanthoma, xanthelasma, or corneal arcus under the age of 50
- aged less than 60 who request screening.

Method

Before a blood test patients will follow a normal diet for three days and then fast for 12 hours.

Results

If serum cholesterol is raised above 6·5 mmol/l the doctor will
- exclude hypothyroidism, diabetes, liver disease, and alcohol abuse
- advise the patient to stop smoking, reduce alcohol intake, and follow a low fat diet
- enter the patient on the disease register.

If the cholesterol is raised above 6·5 mmol/l on repeat testing the doctor will refer the patient to the dietitian.

If the cholesterol is raise above 7·5 mmol/l on repeat testing the doctor will consider lipid lowering drugs if the patient has stopped smoking and has followed a low fat diet.

Aim

The aim of treatment is to achieve a serum cholesterol under 6·6 mmol/l.

Ideas for the preparation and presentation of *needs and deficiencies* are at present crude. We have measures of social need (for example, the Jarman Underprivileged Area Score[13]) but no agreed method of measuring health care need, as opposed to demand.[14] It is perhaps in this area that a patient participation group can be most valuable. It can consider the practice from an external viewpoint, suggesting areas of need and items for improvement. Health visitors and social workers may be able to help. But at the end of the day the practice must decide what particular local needs are to be highlighted and addressed. Some may require political

---

Targets for 1989–90

In last year's report many targets were set; many of these have been achieved. We list the targets we set below, along with new targets that we feel are appropriate.

Targets achieved

To publish another report including more details of our activities

To have a breakdown of cases seen by district nurses

Age breakdown for physiotherapy referrals

Outcome of physiotherapy referrals by condition and doctor

Diagnosis of referrals to physiotherapy according to doctor

Numbers of patients dying at home

New registrations by county

Investigations by type

Night visits and temporary residents seen

Well man and well woman clinic audit

100% call and recall system entries; preventive uptake rates can be identified for all groups

Targets outstanding (may be partly achieved)

Referral patterns to district nurses

Outcome measures in district nursing

Numbers of patients dying at home, divided into terminal care and sudden deaths

Hospital referrals (trainees shown individually)

Investigations, classed by doctor

Measles, mumps, and rubella immunisation rates (not yet 98%)

Cervical cytology (not yet 90% in target groups)

Blood pressure recording—a long way to go to reach 90%

Tetanus immunisation (far short of 80%)

New targets

To finalise protocols of care in major chronic conditions

To audit the protocols

To complete the building of the extension and fully equip it

In preparation for more detailed audits to carry out a patient satisfaction survey

---

action, others social intervention. There will, however, be areas where the practice can act directly to help.

The practice might identify, for example, a high rate of ischaemic heart disease in its area, associated with a low social class structure. It might decide to increase the number of the well person clinics, to set up smokers' groups, and to run a health education initiative on diet. All these initiatives might involve recruiting practice nurses, counsellors, and dieticians.

The practice might additionally decide to campaign for increased health visiting time, improved school meals, increased health education in schools, and a local initiative from the regional health education unit.

For most practices, however, targets are more down to earth. They should include the successes and failures of the targets published a year earlier, and should set new ones for the coming year (see box on page 214). Some targets will be longer term and this should be stated, but an appropriate time scale should be given. It might, for example, be impractical to aspire to new premises in the short term, but these may be a common practice goal. It would be worth stating this with a time label, such as "within five years."

Creating a practice report

Who does the work?

Creating a practice report may at first seem a daunting task. The work, however, is not onerous when split between many members of the team.

The first report can skimp on statistics and concentrate on description. Each member of the team can be asked to write a report on his or her past year, and figures that are available from the family practitioner committee can be added. The advantage of this approach is that it allows a short lead in time from decision to product.

It is then crucial to decide what information is needed for the next report. Many items can be collected by using simple recording sheets; for example, we record our routine hospital referrals by having a monthly grid sheet for each doctor with boxes for speciality and location. Every time our secretary types a letter she ticks a box. She also puts an extra copy of each letter into a separate folder for auditing later.

Information systems like these can involve everybody in the practice, but only a small amount of extra effort is needed from each. The receptionists, for example, record daily our appointments and visits, and then one receptionist enters the total workload on weekly summary sheets.

In our practice one partner is editor of the practice report, the practice manager encourages and cajoles the authors of each section, a preventive care nurse does the preventive care and clinical auditing, and a senior receptionist prepares the routine practice statistics.

Since the data are seen within the practice to be valuable for planning and monitoring, no one resents the time put in and the act of publishing rewards those who have collected the data for their efforts over the year.

Definition of data items

It is important for practices to use the few common definitions in their reports to facilitate interpretation and comparison. To this end, these common definitions should be followed, but a fuller set has been published by Howarth et al.[15]

A fully registered National Health Service patient is someone who is fully registered with the family practitioner committee.

This may sound self evident, but practices using computers often include patients on their list as soon as they hand in their cards and exclude them as soon as it is known that they have moved. In a practice with a high turnover but a static total population this should give approximately the same number of patients, but the time lag means that the identity of these patients may vary by up to 10%. To achieve consistency it is necessary to use the same patient base as the family practitioner committee, and this means that the practice must make retrospective adjustments to the date of registration notified by the committee.

Any grouping of patients by age should specify the date of the grouping (usually the first day of a quarter) and it should include those patients who are of the specified age on the specified date.

If, for example, a practice states in its report that it has 80 children aged 5 and it used these as the denominator for immunisations this could have a number of meanings. It could mean the number of children aged 5 on the first day of the year or at the time

216

of the audit for the report. It could mean all those children who were aged 5 at any point in the year or those who had a fifth birthday in the year. To avoid confusion it is therefore necessary to follow the rule set out above.

Any subgroup may be excluded from a grouping provided the criteria for exclusion are explicit and the data for the whole group are given.

If a practice wishes to give the immunisation rate for children born into the practice (as distinct from those that move in after birth) it is quite at liberty to do so. It should, however, give the figures for all the children and clearly define the exclusion criterion used in working out the figures for the subgroup.

The date entered for a procedure is the date on which it is carried out; the date of a diagnosis is the date when it was first made with reasonable certainty.

This rule means that a blood test, for example, is dated from when the sample is taken, not from when the result is received. A diagnosis is dated from the moment that it is made, not from the date when the patient joined the practice with a pre-existing diagnosis, nor from the date on which the diagnosis was entered in the problem list or disease register.

Age grouped data should normally be presented in single years, in 5 year bands, or aggregates of 5 year bands in the series 0–4, 5–9, 10–14, and so on.

This may be self evident but is easily forgotten when auditing an adult group. There is a strong temptation to lapse into bands of, for example, 36–45, as we did in table 21. Table 22 shows confusing age groupings of 20–40 and 40–60, which should be avoided.

Computers

It is difficult to see how a practice can comply with the new contract without a computer. Surely it will be impossible to be a fund holding practice without one? Although a practice report can, of course, be produced manually, a computer will ease the burden of work, increase the scope, and improve the accuracy of the data.

Computers are of course only as good as the information entered and the program used. Many items—for example, the recording of referrals described earlier—can be quite easily recorded manually but others—for example, prevention uptake rates—are laborious to calculate manually and can be done rapidly and accurately by a computer.

A computer can be used also as a word processor and to generate graphics to help in the presentation of complex data. As clinical computer systems for the generation and presentation of data become widespread it will be easier to retain protocols and to audit them.

The future

Practice reports will become more sophisticated. The reason for this is that the management of the health service will become more complex and the professional requirement for general practitioners to demonstrate quality of care will become more pressing.

As a tool for management and quality demonstration the practice report will increasingly be looked upon as an essential part of primary care. Its scope will increase not in response to a desire for self exhibition but as a way to meet the challenges of an evolving health service.

As the complexity of practice reports increases so will their uniformity. This is not to say that they will become drab, repetitive documents, but that they will contain key tables that can be compared with data from previous years and those from other practices. From this will evolve the concept of area reports.

If a practice is to increase its ability to attract resources it will need to cooperate with other practices in the same area. This will mean aggregating data, and some supplementary mutual data gathering—for example, of patient need. One example is the Newark Information Sharing Project, of which I am coordinator.[16]

In this project five practices based on a country town shared information on patient numbers, prevention, chronic diseases, workload, referrals, and investigations. These data were presented in a report for all the practices. For each area examined the average for all the practices combined, and the ranges, were given so that each could see how it compared with the others.

This non-judgmental confidential approach has proved acceptable and cost effective and may become more common as information becomes more available in practices. Such aggregations will help to identify problems, assess trends, and measure improvements in performance.

The Newark Information Sharing Project was a paper based

exercise; but soon practices may be linked electronically so that they can share information on a regular basis. This will make it possible to compare performances on a continuing basis with collections of similar practices while allowing individual practices to demonstrate the results of efforts in particular areas.

Conclusions

In this chapter I have attempted to define and to justify practice reports. The range of material to be included and how to set about producing a report have been considered. It is of course for each practice to decide how, or whether, to proceed.

It must, however, be observed that we have recently moved from a general practice contract in which clinical performance was determined by doctors to one where the government as the customer has determined standards, especially in prevention. This shift can be ascribed to the profession's unwillingness to evaluate its work critically and to set its own targets openly.

If general practitioners are to avoid ever widening state involvement in clinical areas they will need to change their attitudes to the formulation and presentation of ideas and information. One step, perhaps the major step, along this road is the production of high quality practice reports, and I for one look to the day when they will be part of every practice's activity.

1 Urquhart AS. Practice annual reports. *J Roy Coll Gen Pract* 1987;**37**:148.
2 Wilson A, Jones S, O'Dowd TC. Survey of practice annual reports. *J Roy Coll Gen Pract* 1989;**39**:250–2.
3 Gray DJP. Practice annual reports. In: Gray DJP, Gray JP (eds). *The medical annual* 1985. Bristol: Wright, 1985:2282–300.
4 Metcalfe DHH. Audit in general practice. *Br Med J*, 1989;**299**:1293–4.
5 Keeble BR, Chivers CA, Gray JAM. The practice annual report: post mortem or prescription? *J Roy Coll Gen Pract* 1989;**39**:467–9.
6 Department of Health. *General practice in the National Health Service: the 1990 contract*. London: Department of Health, 1989.
7 Department of Health. *Terms of service for doctors in general practice*. London: Department of Health, 1989.
8 Royal College of General Practitioners. *Report from general practice 23: What sort of doctor?* London: RCGP, 1985.
9 Royal College of General Practitioners. *Guide to assessment for fellowship of the Royal College of General Practitioners*. London: RCGP, 1989.
10 Baker R. *Practice assessment and quality of care*. London: Royal College of General Practitioners, 1988. (Occasional paper 39.)
11 Hart JT. *A new kind of doctor*. London: Merlin Press, 1988:237–41.
12 Black N. Annual reports on public health. *Br Med J* 1989;**299**:1059–60.

13 Pritchard P, ed. *Patient participation in general practice*. London: Royal College of General Practitioners, 1981. (Occasional paper 17.)

14 Jarman B. Identification of underprivileged areas. *Br Med J* 1983;**286**:1705–9.

15 Howarth FP, Maitland JM, Duffus PRS. Standardisation of core data for practice annual reports: a pilot study. *J Roy Coll Gen Pract* 1989;**39**:463–6.

16 Pringle M. *Newark information sharing project: one model for medical audit by peer review*. Newark: Health Trends, in press.

Further reading

Cembrowicz S. How to write a practice annual report. *Br Med J* 1989;**298**:953–4.

Ebbs D. How to prepare a practice report. *Update* 1987:940–3.

Derbyshire Family Practitioner Committee. *Practice report writing*. Derby: Derbyshire FPC, 1989.

Westcott R, Jones RVH (eds). *Information handling in general practice*. London: Croom Helm, 1988.

Appendix A
System of care

Receptionist dispensers

The receptionist dispensers are supervised by the practice manager, Kate Batty, assisted by Pauline, our secretary. They have the sometimes difficult task of being "up front," handling inquiries of every sort from people who may be in varying states of distress. All our surgeries, except the one on Saturday morning (which is for emergencies only), are by appointment. Provision is made to fit in extras who feel they have a more urgent problem. Most are seen at the end of surgery, though the very urgent cases are obviously seen immediately. Patients with appointments are usually seen within 15 minutes of their appointed time. We hope that when this does not happen people will understand it has probably been because of an emergency or someone having a major problem. Confidentiality is a major concern in our practice. With this in mind receptionists do not handle letters or results. Any phone inquiries about results are passed to the doctor concerned.

Dispensing

We dispense for everyone in the practice. We like to feel we give a better service than that offered by a prescribing doctor and chemist. By keeping full drug histories of all our patients we are able to prevent drug interaction problems. The repeat prescribing is fully computerised; this not only saves labour but also streamlines ordering and obtaining supplies.

Our two wholesalers deliver at least once a day and this allows us to obtain even items that are not normally stocked within 24 hours in most cases. Because of the need to order some items and the amount of work involved we do ask for two days' notice for all repeat prescribing whenever possible.

Doctors

The doctors operate an on call rota giving 24 hour cover, seven days a week. Consultations are held on five days a week with an emergency session on Saturday morning. Time is set aside for phone consultations both before and after surgeries. The duty doctor is available out of hours on the same number as in the daytime. A pager is carried so that we can respond rapidly even when we are out visiting.

Nurses

The district nursing sisters are attached to the practice. They are available in the building each weekday morning and Wednesday evening for treatment sessions and some investigations. Their work consists largely of visiting patients referred by the doctors and the hospitals. Occasionally some cases are referred by relatives or the patients themselves. All forms of nursing care are provided, including the comprehensive care of the chronic sick and dying. The district nursing sisters are also involved in well man clinics in Collingham.

The preventive care sister

This sister has been appointed to fill the gaps in the services provided by the district nurses and the health visitor. Her responsibilities largely lie in the field of disease prevention: she is involved in immunisation, well women and well man screening, and screening of the fit elderly. With the new contract it is envisaged that she will take on additional duties, including surveying chronic conditions and initial medical checks on newly registered patients.

The health visitor

The health visitor, Glynne Price, is a nurse with further qualifications whose responsibilities lie largely in the field of prevention with a bias towards using her initiative to educate people to look after themselves and their families. Her responsibilities are not restricted but because we are understaffed it is not always possible for her to be fully comprehensive in her surveillance. Hence her duties in Collingham are concerned mainly with mother and baby welfare up to school age although they include well woman, well man, and elderly screening where possible. Unlike most health visitors she is involved also in counselling within the practice. She is one of the members of the immediate team who also has regular duties outside the practice area.

Midwife

The midwife, Andrea Marks, has a statutory duty to care for, survey, and educate mothers in their antenatal, natal, and immediate postnatal stages. Her duties involve antenatal clinics, some deliveries in hospital under the Domino scheme, and postnatal care at home up to the first 28 days. She is involved also in antenatal relaxation classes. She is also working in another practice outside the Collingham District.

Physiotherapist

Sessions are provided on Monday, Wednesday, and Friday afternoons. Referrals are through the doctors in Collingham or hospital consultants. Treatments may involve exercises, local treatments including heat, short wave, ultrasound and interferential (all essentially soothing treatments that promote healing). There are, too, facilities for some forms of traction. Cases that are referred usually involve some form of sprain or joint condition, but occasionally help can be given for other problems. Recently acupuncture has been added to the range of pain treatments.

School nurse

Penny Macfarlane, the senior nurse, takes over surveillance from the health visitor and is responsible for regular checkups of schoolchildren— usually on school premises. She also runs the hearing assessments within the medical centre using the audiometer. She has been working with the team for two years.

Other workers are involved in caring for the community; they include social workers, speech therapists, community psychiatric nurses, liaison health visitors, etc. To fail to describe their duties is not to diminish them, it is simply that they do not work principally from Collingham.

Appendix B

Collingham and District village care

Village care has found its feet in the past year (1988–89); everyone now seems to know what we do.

People have given their support in so many ways, and for this we are most grateful.

We had three major fund raising events last year:
(1) The first, last October, was for the St Barnabas Hospice. We raised £200 from a cheese and wine evening.

(2) A January coffee morning produced £200 for Dr Simon Baker in Peru. It was a dreadful morning, pouring with rain, but people still supported us.

(3) In June we held an event to raise money for a syringe driver for terminally ill patients. Mrs Hallam opened her home for the occasion; and we raised £1000. We thank her and all those who gave so generously. We now have the syringe driver but hope it will rarely be needed. An electric ear syringe was also purchased out of the £1000. Now the foetal heart detector needs replacing; it was the first item of equipment we raised money for, back in 1982.

We are now endeavouring to improve our transport facilities. We wish we could obtain some funding from Lincolnshire, but it seems unlikely. We could do with twice as many drivers, for an increasing number of calls are being received for this service.

	1987–88	1988–89
Patients carried	1 067	2 041
Mileage covered	10 610	11 160

A good programme of evening meetings has been arranged for 1989–90. They will be held, as usual, in Collingham Library at 7.45 on the fourth Tuesday of the month. There will be talks on a variety of interesting topics.

We thank the members of the committee for their tireless efforts, and also our drivers; but most of all we thank the people who attend our meetings and support our fund raising so generously.

We are grateful to the staff at the Health Centre for their patient help.

BARBARA STOCKS

Index